An Uncertain Cure

Studies in Medical Anthropology

Edited by Mac Marshall

An Uncertain Cure

Living with Leprosy in Brazil

CASSANDRA WHITE

RUTGERS UNIVERSITY PRESS

NEW BRUNSWICK, NEW JERSEY, AND LONDON

LIBRARY OF CONGRESS CATALOGING-IN-PUBLICATION DATA

White, Cassandra.
    An uncertain cure : living with leprosy in Brazil / Cassandra White.
        p. cm.—(Studies in medical anthropology)
    Includes bibliographical references and index.
    ISBN 978-0-8135-4456-4 (hardcover : alk. paper)—ISBN 978-0-8135-4457-1
(pbk. : alk. paper)
    1. Medical anthropology—Brazil. 2. Leprosy—Patients—Brazil. 3. Leprosy—
Transmission—Brazil. 4. Leprosy—Brazil—Public opinion 5. Public opinion—
Brazil. I. Title.
    GN295.6.B6W55 2009
    614.5460981—dc22   2008011252

A British Cataloging-in-Publication record for this book is available from the
British Library.

Visit our Web site: http://rutgerspress.rutgers.edu

Manufactured in the United States of America

CONTENTS

ACKNOWLEDGMENTS

The critical, moral, and financial support for my research on leprosy in Brazil has come from many sources. Grants from the Mellon Foundation and from the International Institute of Education's Fulbright Program provided funding for the majority of the research presented in this book, and a Tulane University Dissertation Writing Fellowship allowed me to formulate and articulate my initial analysis of the research. Grants from the University System of Georgia and the Georgia State University Study Abroad Office to develop a study-abroad program in Brazil helped me maintain ties with the leprosy NGOs and clinics where I conducted research.

I would like to thank Maxine Margolis, Randal Johnson, and Charles Perrone for inspiring me to become a Brazilianist. Thanks to William Balée for his advice and support as my dissertation advisor at Tulane University and to Adeline Masquelier and Victoria Bricker for their comments on earlier versions of some of the work included here. I am grateful to the members of a writing group at Sweet Briar College, who made suggestions on my book proposal, in particular, to Matt Calarco, whose extremely positive comments gave me much-needed confidence in my writing. In the preparation of an early draft of the manuscript, writing coach Esther Erlich assisted immensely with helping me meet personal deadlines. Thanks to Kathryn Kozaitis at Georgia State University; her encouraging words and her insights on agency were invaluable in the final stages of preparing this book. Susan McCombie's perspectives and suggestions on my work have also been influential. Thanks also to Isabella Chan, who provided me with excellent comments on the last draft of the book from the perspective of an advanced undergraduate student.

I would also like to thank anonymous reviewers of several peer-reviewed journals to which I have submitted material based on the research discussed in this book. No significant content in this book has been published elsewhere, but short passages, concepts, and interview excerpts have appeared previously in the journals *Health Education Research*, *Medical Anthropology Quarterly*, *Leprosy Review*, and *História, Ciências, Saúde—Manguinhos*.

I am indebted to Judith Justice, who served as a reviewer for this book and who (in the context of preparing this book and in other communication over the years) has deepened my understanding of the politics of leprosy control at the global level. I am very grateful for her thoughtful comments on my manuscript. I also appreciate Felton Ross's comments on the first chapter. Thanks to Samantha Solimeo, who suggested I submit my proposal to Rutgers University Press. I greatly appreciate the support and advice of my editors at Rutgers, Mac Marshall and Adi Hovav. Suzanne Kellam, production editor at Rutgers, patiently answered my nearly daily e-mails as I worked on my final draft. Thanks also to my amazing copy editor, Brooke Goode. Working with Rutgers Press has been an incredibly positive experience. I accept any responsibility for errors that remain in the book.

Thank you to Julia Elwood and Tanya Thomassie, who welcomed me at the Gillis W. Long Hansen's Disease Center in Carville, Louisiana, and allowed me to collect oral histories there. Thanks also to all of the residents and staff who sat for oral history interviews with me. I learned a great deal about the experience of leprosy and leprosy treatment in the past and present through the narratives I collected at Carville. I am also grateful to José Ramirez, Jr., who gave me permission to use an excerpt of his oral history in this book.

I would like to thank everyone in Brazil who facilitated my research. In particular, I appreciate the help of José Augusto da Costa Nery and Artur Custódio de Sousa, who made my research possible and gave me a more complete understanding of the leprosy situation in Brazil. Thanks also to Denise Vieira, Rita Pereira, Ruth Reis do Amaral, Regina Maria da Cruz, Ismênia Galvão, Margarethe Lutebark, Emília dos Santos, Anna Maria Sales, João Carlos Regazzi Avelleira, and all of the healthcare workers, volunteers, and others I may have forgotten to mention who helped me at different points in my research. Thanks to my Brazilian "sister" Martha Alves and to her family for their friendship and generosity and to Maryse Bacellar, for all her help and kindness over the years.

I would like to thank my parents, Bill and Judy White, who helped cultivate my interest in anthropology (and in learning in general) from the time I was very young. They have continued to be supportive of my career choice, even though it has taken me farther away than they might have liked. Thanks to my in-laws, Arleen and Les Emmons, for their moral support and love over the years. Loving thanks to my husband, Chris de Francisco, who has been my companion in the field and in life for more than a decade and who has come to be a true *carioca*. He has also patiently read drafts of my work and provided much-needed words of encouragement at every stage of my writing. Special thanks to my daughter, Daphne, for her sweetness and her patience in her first year of life, during which I did most of the final editing of this book.

Above all, I must thank all of the individuals affected by leprosy who graciously gave me their time to talk about very personal experiences. This book is dedicated to them. I was amazed by their generosity and openness, and I hope that in some way, the information and illness narratives that these people shared with me will improve treatment for others affected by this disease.

An Uncertain Cure

1

Introduction

Why Leprosy?

"How did you come to study leprosy?"

"Why leprosy?"

"I didn't know it still existed."

"Aren't you afraid of getting it?"

These are some of the typical questions and comments I have heard since 1995, when I started working with people affected by leprosy in Brazil and the United States. In the popular imagination of the West, at least, "leprosy" and the archetypal "leper" are confined to biblical or medieval settings. Even in Brazil, which is second only to India for the highest prevalence of the disease and where over thirty-eight thousand new cases were detected in 2005 (WHO 2007b), awareness among the general public of leprosy's existence is limited. In the United States, most people have heard of or read about the isolation of patients in what were once known as "colonies" or "leprosaria," places like Kalau-papa on the island of Molokai, Hawaii, and Carville in Louisiana. Few, however, are aware that in the twenty-first century, leprosy is still a problem in many countries throughout the world.

Now, after spending more than ten years studying leprosy (also known as Hansen's disease) and working with patients and former patients, it is easy for me to be judgmental about prejudices and pre-conceptions surrounding the disease. Yet before I began focusing on leprosy in Brazil, I had the same stereotypical images of the disease that are held by many in the Western world who are not personally acquainted with it. I assumed that leprosy caused your flesh to rot and your limbs to fall off. I remembered the film *Jesus Christ Superstar* (Jewison 1973) in which the "lepers" ask Jesus to heal them: "See my eyes, I can hardly see/ See my skin, I'm a mass of blood/ See my legs, I can hardly stand," sang the actors, covered from head to toe in white rags as they cried and grasped at Jesus, until he became overwhelmed in a sea of tormented souls. I also recalled the film *Ben Hur* (Wyler 1959), in which the title character's mother and sister are afflicted with leprosy, and people throw stones at them, crying out "Unclean, unclean!" I thought of leprosy as being extremely contagious and quite terrifying; my foremost impression was that it was a disease of the past.

In 1993 I saw a documentary on the A&E network that changed the course of my research and steered my life in a new direction. It was a British production entitled "Thalidomide: Still With Us" (Cutler 1993), dealing with the second generation of children affected by thalidomide syndrome born in recent years in Brazil. Thalidomide produced severe birth defects in thousands of infants worldwide born to women who took the drug during pregnancy in the late 1950s through 1961 (Perri and Hsu 2003). In nearly fifty countries, thalidomide was marketed for the control of morning sickness in pregnant women. The drug causes birth defects, including shortened limbs (a condition known as phocomelia), and other health problems. According to the documentary, in Brazil thalidomide was prescribed for leprosy.

Although I had studied abroad and conducted some research for my MA thesis in Rio de Janeiro, I did not know leprosy was a problem in Brazil. After seeing this documentary, I decided to investigate the use of thalidomide in Brazil from an anthropological perspective. In 1995 I had a chance to return to Brazil to conduct preliminary research. My first day in Rio de Janeiro proved especially fortunate. I stayed with my friend Maryse, a social worker I met on my first trip to Brazil. She lived in the upscale neighborhood of Ipanema, in an apartment with an amazing view of the Lagoa (Lagoon) Rodrigo de Freitas and of Corcovado mountain, topped by the immense Cristo Redentor (Christ the Redeemer) statue. At the time, she was renting a room to a young woman named Glória, a Colombian medical intern and aspiring plastic surgeon. Glória had come to Brazil to work with Ivo Pitanguy, an internationally famous Brazilian plastic surgeon who has operated on celebrities and royalty from all over the world but also performs surgeries free of charge for patients who cannot afford to pay but have life-threatening or life-altering conditions that plastic surgery could alleviate. She laid out a wonderful vision of the transformative potential of plastic surgery and gave me a new perspective on a field of medicine that I had previously thought of as one that was only about profiting from the insecurities and vanities of the wealthy.

Glória offered to introduce me to physicians in the dermatology branch of the downtown hospital where she was interning, Santa Casa de Misericórdia (Holy House of Mercy). Though the physical manifestations of leprosy are on the skin, it is not technically a dermatological condition, but it is often treated at dermatology clinics. When I met the physician in charge, I recognized him immediately, as he was featured in the documentary that had inspired me. Dr. José Augusto Nery, known as Dr. Zé Augusto, was enthusiastic about my research, and in this first meeting at his clinic, I learned that the issues surrounding thalidomide use were more complex than I had imagined.

He introduced me to a middle-aged woman sitting in a tiny exam room. She was in a great deal of pain from "leprosy reaction," a condition commonly associated with leprosy that can cause fever, pain, and nerve damage. Thalidomide is one of the more effective treatments for leprosy reaction. The Brazilian government had passed a law that year (1995) that prohibited women of reproductive age from receiving thalidomide. Instead, this woman was taking a steroid medication, prednisone. This woman was not responding well to the steroids, and steroid medication was more expensive than thalidomide, which was being produced in Brazil and was relatively cheap.

On this preliminary research trip, I met another person in Rio de Janeiro who was to become instrumental to my understanding of the leprosy situation in Brazil—Artur Custódio de Sousa, the coordinator of a nongovernmental organization (NGO) called MORHAN (Movement for the Reintegration of People Affected by Hansen's Disease). MORHAN works to educate the public about leprosy, its treatment, and the stigma surrounding it. It also provides advocacy services for leprosy patients and their families. Artur, then twenty-seven, had worked as a volunteer with leprosy-related issues since he was thirteen, and he had brilliant insights into the problems surrounding leprosy treatment in Brazil. He impressed me with his ideas and energy, and although he did not have a college degree at the time, we discussed Michel Foucault, a philosopher whose work is rarely read outside of academic circles in the United States. He told me about MORHAN's investigations of second-generation thalidomide syndrome cases, of which, according to a more recent article coauthored by Artur, they have identified sixty-one individuals (Oliveira, Bermudez, and Souza 1999). He invited me to attend a meeting of mothers and their children who had disabilities related to thalidomide syndrome. Artur flooded me with information, allowing me to peruse MORHAN's library and view video clips they had collected. He introduced me to volunteers, some of whom were former leprosy patients. Artur assured me that he would give me all the help I needed if I decided to do this research in Rio.

On my return to the United States I mapped out my project, hoping to return to Brazil as soon as possible to carry out the research on patient experiences with leprosy treatment. Life circumstances slowed me down a little, and I did not return to Brazil until 1998. In the meantime, however, a friend in the graduate social work program at Tulane University in New Orleans, where I was a student at the time, told me he knew a young woman who was interning at the Gillis W. Long Hansen's Disease Center in Carville, Louisiana. I contacted her, and a few weeks later, an unexpected research opportunity presented itself.

Carville

It was serendipitous that Carville was so close to where I was living. I learned about Carville, as this former leprosy treatment hospital, confinement center, and community was known, during a phone conversation with a friend who was attending graduate school at Louisiana State University in Baton Rouge. He was out on his motorcycle at night, driving aimlessly, when he came to the dead end of River Road along the Mississippi and saw the entrance to the former leprosarium. From his description of the eerie feelings the place evoked in him, I pictured

dark and gloomy grounds, with forbidding iron gates covered in Spanish moss. Through the gates, I expected to see the crumbling ruins of
structures that once housed America's most unfortunate individuals,
who had committed no crime and yet were forced into isolation from
family and society for the rest of their lives.

The real Carville, however, was nothing like I imagined. There
were no ruins, and in fact, there was a lively community of nearly
160 residents in 1996 (when I first visited). Within the modern gates,
which, I was told, served to keep people out rather than keep patients
in, Carville was beautiful, with wide spaces of farmland dotted with
oak and pecan trees and bright white buildings dating from different
eras. Nancy Hoffer, the social work student from Tulane, took me on
a tour and introduced me to several of the facility's residents, including Betty Martin, author of the best-selling book *Miracle at Carville*
(1950). In 1928, Betty, then a nineteen-year-old New Orleans socialite,
was diagnosed with leprosy and sent to Carville, where she wound up
spending many years of her life, eventually falling in love with another
patient and fleeing the facility, only to come back when his condition
worsened. When the "miracle" of the discovery of sulfone drugs to treat
leprosy happened, Betty and her husband, Harry, left again, though they
later retired to Carville, as it had become home to both of them.

I also met Julia Elwood, a former patient who was, when I met her,
the director of public relations at Carville. She too had been diagnosed
with leprosy as a teenager and spent her high school years at Carville
in the early 1960s. She had many difficult and lonely days there, but she
adapted to community life, serving as Mardi Gras queen, socializing
with other young patients, and working on the staff of *The Star*, a Carville publication edited by patients in residence. Julia had no apparent
signs of having had leprosy, although her life was completely transformed because of a public health policy that required Carville patients
to be isolated during their extended treatment program.

When I met Julia, she was involved—with the help of media specialist Tanya Thomassie—in a project to compile videotaped oral histories
of patients and staff at Carville; the interviews were to be transcribed
and catalogued at the T. Harry Williams Center for Oral History at Louisiana State University libraries. Julia was eager to have some assistance

with this time-consuming project, so she set up some interviews for me and gave me some tapes to transcribe. My first interviewee was a Latina woman who asked to be interviewed in her dorm-style room on the grounds of Carville. Through this interview, I had my first glimpse into the life of a person whose world had been changed dramatically because of leprosy. Over the next two years, visiting Carville once or twice per month, I interviewed thirteen former patients, two physicians, a nun, a Catholic priest, a Protestant minister, and several staff members, some of whom had worked at Carville for decades and some who also had parents who had worked there. For the most part, the life histories of former patients were the most profound and moving, but staff members told fascinating stories about life at Carville as well.

Sadly for many of the workers and residents, Carville was converted into a home for troubled teenagers in 1999. Residents were encouraged to accept a yearly stipend to move away, though a few who had known no other home for decades were allowed to stay. The interviews I collected at Carville provided me with many ideas for my future research in Brazil. Though I have summarized my work at Carville elsewhere (White 1996, 2003), I include in this book some comparisons of the experiences of people with leprosy at Carville and in Brazil. During my work at Carville, through my interviews with physicians and collection of documents and articles from Carville's library, I also learned a great deal about historical and epidemiological aspects of leprosy.

Leprosy: Etiology, Symptoms, History

Many popular beliefs about leprosy are exaggerations or distortions of the biomedical model of the disease. According to the medical model, for example, leprosy does not cause flesh to rot or limbs to fall off; leprosy bacilli can cause nerve damage that can result in lack of sensitivity that leads to injury and, in some cases, secondary infection. Though leprosy is popularly believed to be highly contagious, the biomedical view is generally that its transmissibility is quite low. Anecdotally, at Carville none of the physicians, nurses, or nuns working there ever contracted the disease in the century that it was open. Likewise, I have never met a healthcare worker in Brazil who contracted leprosy, though I met many who worked daily with people who had active cases of the disease. In presenting the biomedical version of leprosy below, I would urge readers to keep in mind that it does not necessarily contain the absolute truth about leprosy. Although the cause of the disease is known, there is still contention within the medical community about everything from exactly how transmission occurs to how individual immunity plays a part in a person's response to the disease (Scollard 2005, 27).

Leprosy is caused by infection with the bacillus (a rod-shaped bacteria) *Mycobacterium leprae*. In its early stages, leprosy symptoms can be quite mild. One of the most common diagnostic symptoms of leprosy is the appearance of one or more lesions or "patches" that tend to be a different color from the rest of the skin. These skin patches can resemble a variety of dermatological conditions, but their characteristic feature is insensitivity. Because these skin patches are not painful, it is common for patients and physicians (particularly those not trained in leprosy diagnosis) to overlook them.

The current biomedical model of leprosy transmission is that it is passed from person to person in liquid droplets emitted during breathing or sneezing. Leprosy bacilli attack the peripheral nervous system and can damage nerve endings, thus causing numbness or a "pins and needles" sensation. After a burn or a cut, for example, a person with nerve damage may not treat the wound; it can thus result in infection, gangrene, and necrosis (tissue death), which in some cases requires amputation. At Carville, I was told the story of a patient who walked all day with a clothespin in his shoe, but because he had lost sensitivity in his feet, he didn't notice it. At the end of the day, the clothespin had cut his foot down to the bone, resulting in permanent damage and disability.

If untreated or undetected in its early stages, leprosy can result in other complications. Some patients develop what is known as "claw hand," in which the fingers become paralyzed in a claw-like position. "Penciling" of the bones in the fingers and toes may occur through bone resorption (a process in which the bone is dissolved and reabsorbed by the body), giving a shrunken and swollen appearance to hands and feet. Carpal tunnel syndrome can occur because of nerve inflammation.

There may be changes to the face and skull in advanced, untreated cases of leprosy due to the action of large concentrations of bacilli, including the destruction of nasal bones and cartilage, which can cause the bridge of the nose to collapse. The deterioration in the nasal area can cause a dramatic alteration in appearance. Concentration of millions of bacilli in the forehead region causes a condition known as leonine facies (literally, lion face) (Hastings 1985; Ortner and Putschar 1985). Ears infiltrated by bacilli may have a bumpy and swollen appearance. Affected individuals may lose their eyebrows and eyelashes. The eyes can be seriously damaged by leprosy, which was, just over a decade ago, a leading cause of blindness worldwide (Brand and Yancey 1993, 143). The bacilli accumulate in the cornea, causing severe damage and the development of cataracts. Leprosy patients in advanced stages of the disease also suffer from anesthesia in their eyes and will rub or touch their eyes without realizing they might be doing damage. They may also experience paralysis of eyelids, which prevents blinking, essential for the eyes to remain clean and moist (143–145).

Some of the complications mentioned above arise during episodes of leprosy reaction, which is a kind of immune response comparable to an allergic reaction to dead leprosy bacilli in the body. Paul Saunderson (2002) estimated that leprosy reaction is experienced by 25 to 30 percent of people with leprosy. Episodes of leprosy reaction are characterized by fever, pain, and inflammation of preexisting skin patches, and they are responsible for much of the nerve damage associated with leprosy. Leprosy reaction may occur before, during, or after treatment (Saunderson 2002). It is common at the initiation of treatment because of the profusion of dead and dying *M. leprae* bacilli in the body, prompting some patients to wonder if their body is responding negatively to the treatment program or having a reaction to medication. Many patients have problems with leprosy reaction for several years after they complete treatment for leprosy, which creates doubts about the curability of the disease for some patients, as will be discussed in more detail below and in subsequent chapters.

Although today there are ways to prevent disabilities associated with leprosy, people who develop severe disabilities before seeking treatment risk permanent disablement. However, physical therapy and proper care of the eyes, hands, and feet can prevent further disability and offer a chance for rehabilitation for some patients. Today there are surgeries available that can improve appearance as well as mobility for leprosy patients. Modern surgical techniques, though available to only a few patients because of the cost, can even rebuild noses and improve mobility in damaged hands and feet.

Leprosy has affected human populations for millennia. Until recently, the disease was thought to have spread from East Asia to the rest of the world, but a comparative study of different contemporary strains of leprosy worldwide indicates either East Africa or Central Asia as likely regions of origin (Grimm 2005). Although there are several historical documents that refer to a disease that may have been leprosy, definitive evidence of its existence comes from the paleopathological record. Leprosy produces visible changes to the skeleton, and current technology allows for DNA analysis of bone and other human remains to determine if leprosy was present. A recently excavated burial site, close to two thousand years old, in the Hinnom Valley of Jerusalem contained the earliest physical evidence to date of the existence of leprosy; the presence of the disease in the remains of an individual was verified by DNA testing (Weizman 2003). Texts in India (Pannikar 1985, cited in Carciániga and Herselman 1999, 158) and China (Gwei-Djen and Needham 1967) that mentioned what could be interpreted as modern leprosy predate this find by six hundred to seven hundred years. The Talmud and the Bible make references to what has been translated as "leprosy," but there is disagreement over what was actually being described. The "leprosy" referred to in the Bible, for example, may have been a general term to refer to a number of different skin conditions, although the disease caused by *M. leprae* may have been among them. "Leprosy" of house walls and of garments is also discussed in the Bible, and this was certainly not an example of a problem caused by *M. leprae*. A third-century B.C.E. Greek translation of the Old Testament used the word *lepra* for the Hebrew word *tzaarath*, and this usage was maintained in a later translation of the Bible into Latin by St. Jerome (Smith 2002).

Throughout Asia and Europe, leprosy (both the disease concept and the scientifically recognized disease caused by the *M. leprae* bacillus) has carried much stigma historically, and people diagnosed with this disease have been persecuted and sometimes isolated from their communities. Severe stigma surrounding leprosy was less common in sub-Saharan Africa. During the colonial era, European missionaries introduced the idea that a degree of shame should be associated with this disease (Vaughan 1991). Some of the roots of leprosy stigma in different parts of the world will be discussed in subsequent chapters.

Dr. Gerhard Amauer Hansen, a Norwegian scientist, discovered the *M. leprae* bacillus in 1873 and suggested that it was the cause of the disease in humans, advancing Louis Pasteur's germ theory (Mange 1992). Hansen himself was convinced that leprosy was extremely contagious (Gussow 1989). Although still considered an infectious-contagious disease, subsequent studies and observations have led leprologists to conclude that prolonged contact with a person transmitting the disease is required for infection. However, leprosy, also known as Hansen's disease, seems to have a great deal to do with an individual's genetic profile and cellular immune system (Scollard 2005). It is estimated that approximately 90 percent of the world's population has a genetic immunity to leprosy (Trautman 1989).

Certain isolated populations that may not have been exposed to leprosy before European contact seem to exhibit greater susceptibility, as in Micronesia and New Guinea (Lewis 1993). For example, leprosy was introduced to the people of the island of Malulu, near New Guinea, in World War II, and by the mid-1950s, 15 percent of the island's population had leprosy. In Hawaii, the first case of leprosy was not diagnosed among the indigenous people until 1835. By 1915, over ten thousand Hawaiians were in leprosy hospitals (Trautman 1989). Other populations seem to have greater immunity to leprosy. Leprosy never took hold among Native American populations. According to Trautman (1989), there is no evidence of a Native American in North America having the disease. On a brief visit to a leprosy referral center in Manaus in the state of Amazonas, Brazil, I learned that there were very few reported cases of leprosy among indigenous populations of the Amazon.

No cure for leprosy was known until the 1940s, when Dr. Guy Faget, at Carville, discovered that sulfone drugs were effective in killing the leprosy bacillus (Stein and Blochman 1963). Monodrug therapy was used for leprosy treatment until 1981, but resistance to dapsone, a sulfone derivative, proved problematic in many patients. In that year, a multidrug therapy (referred to hereafter as MDT) treatment program was introduced that transformed leprosy from a chronic disease requiring lifelong surveillance of the patient to one that could be treated and cured on an outpatient basis. The length of MDT treatment is based on the current classification system used by the World Health Organization (WHO) that separates leprosy into two types: multibacillary (many bacilli) and paucibacillary (fewer bacilli), based on the number of skin lesions. Patients with multibacillary leprosy are thought to have a weaker immune response, resulting in the proliferation of bacilli in their bodies and the subsequent exhalation of large quantities of bacilli, making multibacillary leprosy the contagious form of the disease. In the paucibacillary form, the patient's immune system is somewhat stronger and is able to fight the bacilli to the point where there are relatively few bacilli in the body. People with paucibacillary leprosy are unlikely to transmit the disease to others, according to the current biomedical model. Some scholars have suggested that the division of leprosy into two categories does not reflect the complexity of disease forms and manifestations; earlier classification systems identified up to five different types of leprosy (Scollard 2004).

Multibacillary patients currently receive one year of treatment with an MDT regimen of dapsone, clofazimine, and rifampicin. Paucibacillary patients receive six months of MDT but take only dapsone and rifampicin. When I began my research, multibacillary patients had to remain on MDT for two years and paucibacillary patients for one year, but some studies have shown that one year of treatment is enough (in most patients) to rid the body of all bacilli (WHO 2004). In addition to MDT drugs, patients who experience leprosy reaction generally receive prednisone, thalidomide (for men and women not of childbearing age), and/or clofazimine.

WHO (2007a) reported a 90 percent decrease in prevalence of the disease between 1981 (when MDT was introduced) and 2000. The number of registered cases of leprosy worldwide has dropped from 5.4 million in 1985 (WHO 2007a) to 219,826 at the beginning of 2006 (WHO 2007c). As will be discussed in the final chapter, the reduction in the number of cases may also have to do with how cases are now registered and reported and the reduction in the length of the treatment program. Still, there is no doubt that MDT was a major breakthrough in leprosy treatment, changing the disease from one requiring lifelong treatment to one that could be treated in a much shorter period of time with fewer complications. According to WHO statistics, the incidence, or the number of new cases, of leprosy is also declining. However in 2006, there were still nearly three hundred thousand cases of the disease detected worldwide (WHO 2007b).

Today, leprosy is found primarily in the developing world. Within developing nations, it seems to be most prevalent among the lower socioeconomic segments of the population. Many leprosy researchers believe that poverty contributes to the spread of the disease and to its perpetuation. Diane Lockwood, leprologist and editor of the journal *Leprosy Review*, has suggested that "leprosy should also now be included in the portfolio of diseases associated with poverty and leprosy work incorporated into poverty reduction programmes" (2004, 270). Poverty itself does not cause leprosy, but recent studies have suggested that, in endemic nations or regions, leprosy is associated with certain types of living conditions and with, at the national level, maldistribution of wealth (Lockwood 2004). At the same time, it is important to note that leprosy is not strictly a "disease of the poor": anyone with a genetic susceptibility who is exposed to the disease for a prolonged period can become infected. In endemic nations, there are certainly cases of leprosy among people of the middle and upper classes, but for the most part, these patients often seek treatment with private physicians and their cases go unreported. However, the conditions of poverty may create more opportunities for the disease to spread (Cunha, Rodrigues, and Duppre 2004). Throughout this book, I refer to the role played by structural factors in the continued existence of leprosy and in the experiences of individuals affected by leprosy.

Getting Back to Brazil

At Carville, most of the former patients I met had been diagnosed with leprosy before the development of MDT. Though cured of the disease, their lives had been irrevocably altered by leprosy because of disability, government policies of forced isolation, and/or societal stigma. I returned to Rio de Janeiro in September of 1998, hoping to learn more about the contemporary experience of this disease and its outpatient treatment. My research in Brazil can be described as multi-sited ethnography, or ethnographic research in which the researcher works in multiple settings, is exposed to a variety of perspectives, and attempts to understand how the data fit into a larger spatial and temporal framework (Marcus 1995). Most of my data were collected in the greater metropolitan area of Rio de Janeiro (which includes several satellite municipalities), but I divided my time among multiple activities at different types of locations, including public health posts, the offices of MORHAN, the grounds of a former leprosarium, and a public school adjacent to a favela community. I interviewed a nurse at the Instituto Alfredo da Matta, which houses a leprosy referral center in Manaus, Amazonas. Each piece of information I collected about leprosy in Brazil was compared with data collected from other sources to provide a more holistic and informed view of patients' experiences with this disease.

Participant observation, a cornerstone of anthropological research, was an important component of my work, though it was not carried out in the traditional sense of living among the people one is studying and experiencing everyday life as they do. The "community" of people undergoing outpatient treatment for leprosy is a disparate one. Instead, because I became most interested in the experience of treatment, my participant observation took place largely in referral centers where leprosy was treated. In comparison with many of the other health posts around the city, at these facilities, resources (in terms of medications, supplies, and diagnostic testing equipment) were ample, and physicians and healthcare workers were relatively well paid. Patients were generally pleased with how they were treated at these clinics and sometimes commented to me on the stark contrast between these referral centers and other health posts they had visited. As a reviewer for a journal article I submitted observed, this may be because healthcare workers, particularly physicians, who work with leprosy have typically dedicated their lives' work to this disease, choosing to work in public health facilities over some form of private practice. The warm atmosphere at these referral centers proved amenable to my research:

patients trusted the healthcare professionals who worked there, and, in turn, I was well received.

I spent most of my time at a referral center that served primarily patients who lived in the industrial Zona Norte (North Zone) of the city of Rio de Janeiro and in the working-class suburban municipalities of the Baixada Fluminense (literally, lowland floodplain) to the north of the city. I have decided to keep the name of this facility anonymous to protect the identities of the people I describe. On the days I spent at this clinic, I would typically accompany patients through their clinic visits. I had a chance to observe and converse with patients while they were waiting for their appointments, undergoing diagnostic testing, receiving their diagnosis of leprosy, being counseled by a social worker, taking supervised doses of medication, being examined by interns and physicians, and working with a physical therapist. Many of the patients I interviewed had completed MDT and were there for treatment of leprosy reaction. Over the course of the year I spent in Brazil, I took fieldnotes on the clinic visits of 144 separate patients, several of whom I had the chance to see more than once.

This referral center was also the location where I was able to recruit individuals affected by this disease for in-depth interviews. I prepared detailed interview questions (Appendix A), designed to elicit what Arthur Kleinman (1988) refers to as "illness narratives." In the collection of an illness narrative, the researcher (or health practitioner) looks at the illness, or how the patient experiences a disease within his or her family, culture, and society. Illness, then, is distinguished from disease, which is "what the practitioner creates in the recasting of illness in terms of theories of disorder" (Kleinman 1988, 3) or "the problem from the practitioner's perspective" (5). In the illness narrative interviews I conducted, I attempted to collect snapshots of patients' lives with a focus on the time period beginning when the first symptoms of leprosy appeared until the time of the interview. I interviewed forty-one people who had been diagnosed with leprosy and two others who were being tested for leprosy but who had not yet received a definitive diagnosis. I asked questions about every aspect of the disease process as well as about their background, domestic situation, social activities, employment, and neighborhood. These interviews were tape-recorded and transcribed, with the exception of one individual who preferred that I take notes rather than tape her interview. I conducted most of the patient interviews in available, private spaces at the referral center, including unused examination rooms and an empty classroom in a separate building. All patient names in this book are pseudonyms.

I also interviewed fourteen people who work with leprosy in various capacities. These included physicians, nurses, social workers, psychologists, a physical therapist, a municipal government official, and NGO volunteers. I asked questions from a basic schedule (see Appendix B) that was expanded and tailored to each person according to their position and, in part, to my prior knowledge of their experiences with leprosy. I had worked with most of the individuals I interviewed for several months before conducting a formal interview. In addition to these interviews, I took extensive fieldnotes on numerous informal interviews and conversations held with healthcare workers, volunteers, and people affected by leprosy.

Although I had a good grasp of conversational Brazilian Portuguese upon arriving in Rio, it took some time to learn the many slang terms and colloquial expressions commonly used in Rio and among my working-class sample. I used some interviewing strategies described by Charles Briggs (1986), including drawing on local speech forms to inform the interview questions. Most of the patients interviewed were from Rio de Janeiro and spoke a *carioca* (from Rio) dialect of Brazilian Portuguese, quite different in some aspects of pronunciation and vocabulary from other dialects, such as *paulista* (from São Paulo) and *nordestino* (from the Brazilian Northeast). There were also numerous forms of body language to be aware of, both in the context of interviews and in everyday life in Brazil. "Air kissing" on both cheeks upon friendly greeting and farewell (for men-women and women-women interactions) is the custom in Rio. Doctors and patients did not greet in this fashion because this was reserved for more informal and less hierarchical relationships, although I used it often with patients whom I had interviewed when I saw them on return visits. In Brazil, touching indicates caring or friendship. Touch can also be important in working with leprosy patients in different cultural contexts. In my research at Carville, some residents would not readily offer their hand for shaking, fearing the other person's discomfort, but they were appreciative of a handshake if offered. I found this to be true in Brazil also. This form of touch conveys the message that one views the patient as a normal person, not someone to be feared or avoided.

I also learned certain medical terms and idioms that are used both in a clinical setting and popularly, when talking about leprosy. There were several terms that patients used regularly to describe their symptoms and physical experiences, such as itching, burning, numbness, swelling, pain, and aches. *Formigando* (ants crawling) is a common term for a tingling sensation in the hands due to nerve damage. I quickly learned that *alta* not only means "tall" or "high" in Portuguese but also refers to being discharged or completing treatment. I also learned early on that the lesions, spots, or skin discoloration resulting from leprosy are referred to as *manchas*, the same word that is used in Portuguese for spots or lesions from other skin ailments, including fungus and allergy rashes, and for clothing stains.

Briggs (1986) outlines steps researchers can take to gain competence in "metacommunication," or understanding the unspoken meanings that accompany certain forms of discourse and are implicit in the settings in which speech take place. I tried to be aware of the bias of the setting I chose for the interviews. Because most interviews took place at a leprosy treatment center, there was the risk that patients would see the interview in hierarchical terms, with me in the role of a healthcare professional, which I am not. In pre-interview conversation, I emphasized the fact that I was a student studying social and cultural aspects of disease and that I was not a physician. I was also worried that patients might be afraid to answer questions or complain about physicians or healthcare workers because of my apparent association with the clinic. However, I also asked patients questions about experiences they had had at other clinics or health posts, so they would feel comfortable responding openly, without fear of repercussions.

Another aspect of my research in Brazil consisted of attending self-help-group (*grupo de auto-ajuda*) meetings and informational "waiting room" meetings (*reuniões de sala de espera*) for patients in health posts in the greater metropolitan area of Rio de Janeiro. I attended two self-help-group meetings that were organized by MORHAN volunteers with backgrounds in psychology, social work, and nursing. These meetings were intended for people affected by leprosy and their families and were held in a spacious room that was part of a health post in a municipality just outside of Rio's city limits. I also attended six "waiting room" meetings, educational sessions about leprosy that drew on patients in a large waiting room of a referral center for leprosy where patients with general dermatological problems were also treated. This health post was on the grounds of a former leprosarium; patient fears associated with the facility had prompted healthcare workers and social workers to hold these educational meetings, which consisted of discussions of biomedical views of leprosy as well as popular beliefs held by patients. At both types of meetings, I made observations, participated in discussions, and took notes (after the meeting, so as not to make participants nervous).

From the beginning of my research on leprosy in Brazil to the present, I have worked closely with MORHAN. I use the name of this NGO in this book because the activities I describe and the opinions of MORHAN's representatives are very well publicized in Brazil. I attended informational and educational activities in which they participated, including one *panfletagem*, or event, in which they distributed pamphlets about leprosy and about MORHAN and its services. I made use of their library and their database on phone calls to Telehansen, a line available for the public to call in to ask questions about leprosy and its treatment. This analysis of Telehansen records complemented other sources of information about popular beliefs about leprosy in Rio de Janeiro. On one occasion, I accompanied MORHAN volunteers to a lecture and puppet show about leprosy they gave at a public school in a rural area of Rio de Janeiro state. I also served as an English-speaking liaison for MORHAN, occasionally translating documents, working with them on a WHO grant proposal, and meeting a British cargo ship bringing donated braces and crutches.

Another locus of my research activity was a public school adjacent to a favela community in the Zona Sul, or South Zone, of Rio, which includes the wealthy beach communities of Copacabana and Ipanema. Although there are several favelas on the hillsides of the Zona Sul, leprosy is not common in this part of the city. The favela and school were just a few blocks from the apartment where I lived, and after accepting an invitation to observe an art class taught by a Brazilian friend, I visited the school and talked with some of the school officials. They suggested that I attend some meetings that were mandatory for parents to receive tickets for a *cesta básica*, a government-sponsored package of basic food and household cleaning products, supposedly enough to supply a family of four for a month (Deutsche-Welle 2004). I presented short talks at these meetings and asked parents questions about leprosy (*lepra*) and Hansen's disease (*hanseníase*) in order to understand more about popular ideas about the disease among people who were not affected (or who had not been diagnosed) with the disease.

Although the bulk of my research was conducted in 1998 and 1999, several return trips to Brazil have deepened my understanding of the leprosy situation there. In 2002 I attended the Sixteenth International Leprosy Congress in Salvador, Brazil, and reconnected with several of the physicians, social workers, and nurses I met during my initial period of fieldwork. I also met leprosy researchers from all over Brazil and the world. Several branches of MORHAN were represented at these meetings, and I met many volunteers and former patients. In 2004 I returned to Rio to set up a study-abroad program/anthropology field school for students at Georgia State University. In 2005 and 2006, I coordinated visits for students attending this field school to an outpatient clinic for leprosy in Rio. Artur Custódio de Sousa, of MORHAN, and Dr. Zé Augusto have both guest lectured to my students. In addition to my work in Brazil, other experiences have informed my thoughts about leprosy as presented in this book. In 2002, I had a chance to visit the offices of LEPRA, a leprosy NGO in Colchester, England, to present my work. People who work with stigmatized conditions (including many who work with leprosy) worldwide convened at the 2004 International Workshop on Health-Related Stigma I attended in Soesterberg, Holland. This workshop provided me with new perspectives on my research in Brazil.

Being Flexible

When anthropologists arrive in the field, they often find that their original research questions are not relevant or the methods they intended to use are not feasible. Plans that sound good on paper are not always practical, and although preliminary studies and site visits can help clarify research goals, circumstances may change by the time the study is carried out. Sometimes researchers find their project is more tedious or burdensome than they had anticipated. Although I never got bored with my research topic or needed to dramatically change my research direction, not all of my research plans were realized. For example, I initially planned to focus my research on patient compliance with leprosy treatment and to look at the reasons why patients abandon treatment. Upon beginning my fieldwork, an obvious (at least in retrospect) flaw in this plan became apparent. Patients who had abandoned treatment were not easy to locate because they were no longer coming in to the health posts, and their names and addresses were not retained in health post registries indefinitely. Later in my fieldwork I discovered, in the course of home visits I made with a social worker to *resgatar* (recover) patients who had abandoned treatment, that many had moved, were unavailable, or in some cases, had passed away. I also learned from many healthcare workers and volunteers to whom I spoke early on in my research that abandonment of treatment did not fully explain why leprosy continues to spread in Brazil: late detection of the disease was as, if not more, important. As I began spending time observing at the health posts, I decided that I would take a more inductive approach and allow themes to emerge from the data. Eventually, I came to focus on the explanatory models of patients with regard to different stages of their illness and of their treatment program. I also became interested in the problems patients encountered in seeking a diagnosis and a cure.

I also had to be flexible in my methodology. I had hoped to identify patient interviewees using a valid statistical sampling method. However, several factors made that method of choosing interview participants difficult. Patient records were not available in list form, and contacting patients for interviews using the records at the public health posts did not prove fruitful. A social worker who was very enthusiastic about my project agreed to send aerograms or postcards through the mail to individuals who she deemed to be interesting interviewees because they had particularly complex case histories. Many Brazilians in the lower socioeconomic stratum have no home telephones (though today, most

Brazilians have cell phones). At that time, sending aerograms (each with a prepaid return postcard) was one of the most convenient ways for clinics to keep in touch with patients. However, the aerogram method was not successful for setting up interviews. Some patients responded positively, saying they would arrive at the clinic on the date and time suggested by the postcard, but only one interview participant actually showed up on the expected day during the first few attempts at this form of recruitment. Even though the social worker coordinated the interview date with the date of the patient's scheduled appointment, patients were not always able to come to their appointments for a variety of practical reasons (such as work, transportation issues, and problems at home). They may also have been wary of being interviewed.

I found that the best way to recruit patients for interviews was through convenience or haphazard sampling (Bernard 2002, 184). I interviewed patients who were willing and able to be interviewed as they came in for their appointments at the public health post. Certainly, this interview selection process was biased. Not all patients I met could be interviewed. Many patients who came in were experiencing leprosy reaction and were in too much physical distress to sit for an interview. Others had to have several tests done following their appointment or had to leave immediately afterwards to go to work. However, because many patients returned once or twice per month, I was able to interview some of them on their return visit. Essentially, it was up to me to take the initiative to ask a patient if he or she would be interviewed, although occasionally a physician or social worker would point out a particular patient who they thought would make a good interview participant (also introducing bias, as they chose patients who were having more problems with the disease than the norm). At times I also used judgment sampling (182), since I sometimes chose patients who seemed as though they had a story to tell, based on informal conversations.

Although I was not able to obtain a random sample, I felt that my interviews provided valuable and significant data about the experience of leprosy in Rio de Janeiro. The results of my interviews with patients formed only a part of a larger body of information I collected in Brazil. Each experience or model held by leprosy patients I interviewed was triangulated with information based on observations from my other primary forms of data collection and observation as well as from secondary sources of information. For example, only one patient mentioned that she had to buy one of the medications that is supposed to be provided free of charge to leprosy patients. I could not use her experience to make any statements about access to medications in Brazil, but I incorporated her claim into future interview questions with individuals who might give me more information on the subject. I found out from an interview with a health official that this was not a problem in the municipality of Rio de Janeiro but that other nearby cities had problems with distribution and supply of this medication. I also discussed this issue with representatives of MORHAN, who confirmed that a lack of essential medications sometimes occurs in some of the more remote regions of Brazil and in municipalities outside of Rio de Janeiro. From this one patient's experience, I was able to explore new topics with people who have extensive experience working with leprosy and to identify a problem that many patients might experience in Brazil.

Theoretical Underpinnings

An oft-treated subject in medical anthropology is the relationship between the patient and the clinical biomedical world (e.g., the Western medical tradition) and how this relationship fails many patients in its lack of a holistic perspective. A holistic approach to illness takes into account all aspects of a patient's life, including family life, work situation, ethnic background, socioeconomic status, and gender roles; the person's "whole" life is analyzed in a holistic approach. Biomedical practice is based on the principle of the separation of mind and body as proposed by sixteenth-century philosopher René Descartes. This so-called "Cartesian dualism" has been useful to scientists and physicians in terms of looking at the human body as a machine with interconnected parts that function properly or break down because of observable phenomena. However, physicians trained in the Western biomedical system sometimes discount less tangible sources of illness complication, such as those that are external to the patient, as well as those that may arise from a connection between the mind and the body (Scheper-Hughes and Lock 1987). Although healthcare workers do not universally see patients simply as objects of study or examination, the focus of biomedicine has traditionally been the physical body and its ailments rather than the patient's social environment. Medical anthropologists seek to understand disease from a broader perspective, looking at how the patient's experience of disease is shaped by his or her cultural and socioeconomic background and daily reality.

As mentioned above, the work of anthropologist and psychiatrist Arthur Kleinman discussed the ways that physicians often reinterpret, and in the process, sometimes misinterpret, the words of patients, in the interest of diagnosing and treating a disease. Kleinman (1988) noted the importance of listening to patients and understanding their words in the context of the particular culture or subculture of which they are a part. His emphasis on the validity of the narratives and explanatory models of patients in discussing their illnesses was instrumental in my formulation of a theoretical perspective and of the primary project methodology of collecting patients' stories about different aspects of leprosy and leprosy treatment.

One aspect of patients' experiences with leprosy treatment has to do with the choices patients have in treatment options. Several authors have treated the subject of medical pluralism. The decision-making process for patients and their families in regions where there are numerous paradigms for explaining and treating illness has been described by Libbet Crandon-Malamud (1993) in the ethnography *From the Fat of Our Souls*. She wrote about how the choices of Aymara and mestizo peasants in a small highland village in Bolivia reflect their desires to belong to a particular group or to improve or change their status in society. Bruce Kapferer, in his *A Celebration of Demons* (1983), a fascinating ethnography about demon exorcism as healing in Sri Lanka, has also written about the pluralistic system in place there and of the numerous specialists and healers consulted for illnesses. An exorcist is consulted for an illness only after patients had consulted a biomedical physician, an Ayurvedic physician, and an astrologer, with some patients having also visited Buddhist monks or deity shrines (56). Understanding medical pluralism and attempting to interpret why people make the choices they do was important to my research in Rio de Janeiro, where people employ numerous forms of healing

alternative to biomedicine, including various forms of religious healing and home remedies.

Cognitive anthropology is another helpful theoretical tool in the
identification of popular meanings of disease and folk models of leprosy in Brazil. While people in every culture are born with a comparable
range of cognitive capacities, culture and environment shape perception into a particular form. Within cognitive anthropology, ethnoscience focuses on how people in different cultures categorize aspects of
the world around them. Ethnoscience is based on the idea that "real
culture exists only in the minds of the culture bearers" (Garbarino
1977, 82). It can be used to study the ways in which things in the physical world are named and categorized in a particular society. Ethnoscience may include learning the local names or classification systems
for animals, plants, colors, physical features of the landscape, people,
illnesses, and medicines. Contrasting folk or popular classifications of
leprosy with scientific classifications allowed me to identify potential
conflicts in communication between physicians and patients. Learning
the local terms and corresponding definitions of the words *lepra* and
hanseníase in Brazil was also vital to an understanding of how patients
would respond to diagnosis and treatment.

Phenomenology is also useful in attempting to understand individual experiences of illness. Phenomenology is essentially the idea that a
person's experience of something (illness, pain, pleasure) is the most
valid version of reality there can be. Martin Heidegger (1962) proposed
that subjective experience is real to the individual and therefore constitutes an important reality. How a person with leprosy feels or says they
feel should be an indication for physicians of how "well" or "unwell"
they are, regardless of whether or not they are technically "cured" of
leprosy. Marilda Andrade, a nurse I met with in Brazil who has worked
extensively with leprosy patients in Rio de Janeiro, wrote her PhD dissertation on the conflict surrounding patients' understanding of the
cure for leprosy (1997). As mentioned above, a patient is considered
"cured" after six doses of the standard treatment for paucibacillary
patients (fewer than five lesions) and twelve doses for multibacillary
patients (five or more lesions). However, patients often experience
problems related to leprosy for years after treatment is complete.

Although the bacilli in the body may be dead, the patient may have irreversible disability and require treatment for leprosy reaction for years after the physician has declared the patient "cured." Essentially, the physician's declaration of a patient as "cured" means nothing to a patient who is still undergoing problems that he or she relates to leprosy. A phenomenological approach can also be understood as an emphasis on the emic model of understanding. In anthropological research, the *emic* perspective is that of the people in the culture one is researching, while the *etic* perspective is that of the observer or outsider. For example, many people in Brazil think that leprosy comes from dogs and many other sources, to be discussed in chapter 3: this is an emic model. By contrast, the etic model, in this case the biomedical model, posits that the leprosy bacillus is transmitted through droplets emitted by contagious individuals when breathing.

World-system theory, or analysis, as posited by Immanuel Wallerstein (1974) and elaborated by Eric Wolf (1982) and Sidney Mintz (1985), supplies another theoretical component to this project. In world-system theory, situations, events, and conflicts can be understood as products of a series of political and economic events across time and space rather than as isolated phenomena. In particular, Wallerstein emphasized the system of capitalism and commodity production that emerged under European colonialism and has influenced cultures and economies on a global level. Mintz, in his excellent book *Sweetness and Power*, illustrated how the rise to prominence of sugar as an important part of the British and later American diet was dependent on colonialism, the trans-Atlantic slave trade, and the Industrial Revolution. Although leprosy is not a commodity, the history of leprosy in Brazil can be analyzed in the same way that Mintz looked at sugar. As I will discuss in more depth in chapter 2, the existence of leprosy in Brazil can be traced to Portuguese expansion in the New World, the importation of enslaved West Africans, and capitalist development which involved a number of boom-and-bust economic cycles in Brazilian history. Its perpetuation in Brazil can partly be understood in terms of the maldistribution of wealth in modern Brazil and Brazil's status in the global economy.

World-system theory fits in well with critical medical anthropology, which stresses the importance of understanding how political, socioeconomic, cultural, and historical circumstances impact health beliefs and medical systems. Government policies and biomedical discourse related to leprosy are also heavily influenced by such circumstances. A few social scientists (Gussow 1989; Justice 1995; Vaughan 1991) have shown how leprosy treatment and stigma through history can be connected to synchronous events or situations. Their observations resemble those of Michel Foucault (1994) in his detailed analysis of how theories of disease, medicine, and the body in late eighteenth-century France paralleled the sociopolitical atmosphere of the time. Foucault (1988) also explicitly discussed this phenomenon in relation to political decisions about how to handle people diagnosed with leprosy during the Middle Ages and how the established facilities, or leprosaria, were later filled with those culturally defined as "insane."

Discussions of how diseases and their treatments change through time have been put forward by many. For example, John Gabbay (1982), writing about how asthma has been understood in the Western medical tradition over the past few centuries, pointed out that in the 1920s, tobacco was used as a treatment for asthma in patients who previously were nonsmokers, whereas today smoking tobacco is often seen as a potential contributor to this disease. Essayist Susan Sontag (1990) noted that tuberculosis, which was at one time seen as a romantic disease to which only those with a sensitive, artistic demeanor were susceptible, has come to be seen primarily as a disease of the poor. Sontag also observed how stigmatizing attitudes about cancer decreased remarkably toward the end of the twentieth century, to be replaced by HIV/AIDS as a taboo disease. Similarly, Emily Martin (1994) analyzed changes in theories of contagion and immunity that reflect trends and events in history and popular culture in the United States during the second half of the twentieth century. Martin's observations of how immunity is understood are particularly relevant to a study of leprosy, since both popular and biomedical perceptions of its contagion alter with the political climate.

Finally, I draw on the literature on structural violence to explore reasons why leprosy has not yet been eradicated and to understand problems individual patients experience before and during treatment. Peace activist Johan Galtung described structural violence as violence that is "built into structure" (1969, 171), such as the structure of a highly stratified society or one in which certain forms of discrimination or hegemony are entrenched. Many anthropologists and other social scientists view structural inequalities as causing many of the world's problems for which the poor often received misplaced blame. Philippe Bourgois (1995), for example, noted how historical and contemporary structural factors set the stage for the prevalence of crack dealing among young men in East Harlem. Similarly, Donna Goldstein (2003) discussed how the nature of the class system in Brazil contributes to structural violence that affects the standard of living for people in the favelas of Rio de Janeiro. The analysis of structural factors as they relate to health issues can be used in conjunction with a world system and critical medical anthropological approach. Nancy Scheper-Hughes (1992) and Paul Farmer (1993, 1999) have written about the effects of structural violence on the mental and physical health of the poor in the Brazilian Northeast and in Haiti, respectively. In Brazil, where hierarchy and paternalism are powerful forces in the culture, illness can both reflect and reinforce some of the power struggles that people experience on a daily basis. Farmer (1999, 2004) has been most vocal, in recent years, about the proliferation of many infectious diseases, including tuberculosis and HIV/AIDS, as an example of structural violence. With leprosy, one can point to the proximate causes, such as the *M. leprae* bacillus or prolonged exposure to a contagious individual, but a more holistic approach takes into account the underlying reasons why leprosy might be prevalent in a particular part of the world in the first place, how living conditions contribute to the spread of the disease, and how patient agency is limited directly and indirectly by economic inequalities.

Agency in Treatment-Seeking Behavior

An emerging theoretical concept within the social sciences is the idea that people are not mere victims of larger historical, socioeconomic, and political forces, but rather are (or have the potential to be) creative forces in shaping their own futures and destinies. People have agency, or, as anthropologist Laura Ahearn (2001, 112) defines it, "the socioculturally mediated capacity to act." Humans are capable of making individual choices and of taking action using the tools at their disposal or, in some cases, seeking out new tools and ideas they can use for this purpose. However, the actions that people take may be limited by the reality of their daily lives if their access to economic resources, social capital, and cultural capital (Bourdieu 1986) is likewise limited by structural inequalities (Farmer 1999).

In the case of people affected by leprosy in Brazil, I found that individual agency played a much larger role in patients' treatment-seeking behavior than I had initially thought in what, in hindsight, were my naïve early impressions. Before I began my research, informal discussions with people who worked in various capacities with working-class Brazilian patients led me to consider people among this socioeconomic class as fatalistic in their approach to health. There is an element of fatalism in Brazilian culture in general, reflected in the commonly uttered phrases *se Deus quiser* (God willing) and *a vida é assim* (that's life). In the song "Tlmoneiro" (Helmsman), Paulinho da Viola, a renowned samba artist, sings: *Não sou eu que me navega, quem me navega é o mar* (It's not me who navigates [my life], who navigates me is the sea) (Viola and Carvalho 1996). The narrator of the song describes a difficult life in which he is carried along by the waves and by God.

In fieldnotes I took during my preliminary research project, I speculated that this fatalism had to do with "the poor's sense of lack of control over their own lives—they are controlled, manipulated by the government, their employers, doctors as well. Thus, when they are given instructions to take specific medicines, do specific actions to protect their bodies, there may be a block—a psychological barrier—to carrying out these instructions independently. They are accustomed to suffering and perhaps do not make the connection between following doctors' orders carefully and relieving physical discomfort" (June 4, 1995). Based on my subsequent fieldwork with leprosy patients, I came to have a decidedly different view. It is certainly true that those in the lower socioeconomic stratum of Brazilian society have fewer options in terms of what they can do to create opportunities for themselves. However, as I began to have extended conversations with people who were in treatment or had completed treatment for leprosy, I did not encounter passive acceptance of leprosy or of suffering. Instead, these were people who not only cared about getting better but who were actively engaged in the process of returning to wellness. Most of them had gone to great lengths to seek a diagnosis, and once they found out what they had, they became participants in restoring their own health.

Although patients did not always do exactly what healthcare professionals instructed them to do, the reasons did not stem from fatalism or lack of engagement but in most cases were related to variables over which they had little or no control. Poverty set the stage for many of the problems that patients faced in their day-to-day lives and in their quest to get well. Problems that arise within the medical encounter, some of which have to do with structural inequalities in Brazilian society, were to blame for some of the problems that patients encountered while in treatment for leprosy. Everyday life for people in the favelas and other low-income communities is much more challenging than for those in the middle and upper classes in Brazil, but the patients I interviewed still aspired to have disease-free, happy lives, and they drew on the resources they had or were provided with to minimize suffering for themselves and their families. In this book, I will discuss some of the structural factors that both limit patient agency and are responsible for leprosy's continued prevalence in Brazil, and I will demonstrate that given the appropriate resources, support, and information, patients' agentive efforts at getting well are more likely to be realized.

2

"Caminhando contra o vento" (Walking against the wind)

Low-Income Living and Leprosy in Rio de Janeiro

The title of the chapter is taken from the Caetano Veloso song "Alegria, Alegria" (Happiness, Happiness) written in 1967 and a well-known (in Brazil) anthem of the *Tropicalismo* (Tropicalism) movement, the songs of which challenged musical styles of the era and formed subtle or not-so-subtle protests of the military dictatorship; as Veloso wrote in his autobiography, *Tropical Truth*, the artists who made up this movement "wanted the freedom to move beyond the automatic ties with the Left and at the same time to account for the visceral rebellion against the abysmal disparities that tear a people asunder" (2002, 6). When it was written, "Alegria, Alegria" was more a commentary on the changing times and the influence of Westernized culture on Brazilian society as well as what ethnomusicologist Christopher Dunn (2001, 66–67) called the "confusing and fragmented experience of urban life" than it was a direct protest of the dictatorship. The first time I heard the song was in 1992, when I was living with a Rio de Janeiro family as a study abroad student; I heard it nearly every day, as it was used as the opening song for the mini-series/soap opera (*novela*) *Anos Rebeldes* (Rebel Years). I came to associate the song with the student movement—university students who marched and protested against the repression of the dictatorship and who were sometimes imprisoned and tortured. Dunn (206) has noted that when this novela aired, "'Alegria, Alegria' was revived as a protest song by middle-class urban youth who took to the streets to denounce a corruption scandal involving [then President] Fernando Collor de Melo," who was later impeached.

My interpretation of the song, then, perhaps distorts its original meaning and is colored by my first visit to Brazil, my first experience of seeing so much that is wonderful and so much that is sad about this nation. For me, this song has always brought to mind the frustration of millions of Brazilians who, in encountering the extreme bureaucratic workings of society, the harsh poverty of everyday life, racism, and a glass ceiling of educational opportunity and social mobility, feel like they are walking, as the song says, "*contra o vento, sem lenço, sem documento*" (against the wind, without a handkerchief, without documents), or, as Caetano Veloso (2002,108) wrote, "the documentation relentlessly required by the state." Daily life for the majority of Brazilians who are not among the ranks of the economic elite can be extremely challenging. As mentioned in chapter 1, the people I interviewed who were affected by leprosy lived in favela communities, in low-income government housing, or in lower-middle-class homes or apartments, primarily in the Zona Norte of Rio and in outlying municipalities of the Baixada Fluminense, such as Nova Iguaçu, Belford Roxo, and Duque de Caxias. In my interviews, I asked several questions that helped me get a better picture of the problems of everyday life. Visits to several favelas and to the Baixada during the course of my research and since have given me more direct knowledge of these communities. Before beginning my research, I hypothesized that the hardships of everyday life for patients among Rio's lower and lower-middle economic classes might make leprosy less than a central concern. To some extent, this was true, particularly because leprosy is not life-threatening and because many of the severe disabilities associated with it in the past are preventable. But for people I met whose health, social life, and work situation had changed because of the disease, leprosy tended to exacerbate the problems of being poor in this Brazilian megacity, and most patients were eager to seek a cure for their illness. Patients' illness experiences were inextricably linked to their living conditions and socioeconomic status.

In addition to making daily life difficult for the patients I met, the Brazilian socioeconomic system also contributes to the perpetuation of leprosy in Brazil. Brazil's wealth distribution is among the most uneven worldwide, with the richest 20 percent of the population earning 64 percent of the country's income and the poorest 20 percent earning only 2.2 percent of the income (World Bank 2002). While the middle- and upper-class lifestyle and standard of living in Brazil is not unlike that in the U.S. or Europe, a large percentage of the population (47.2 percent in 1999) does not have access to sewers, and 23 percent (not including those in rural regions of states in the Amazon basin region) do not have running water (IBGE 2000). A brief look at the history of leprosy in Brazil, which runs parallel to Portuguese conquest, colonialism, slavery, and its aftermath in the "New World," provides a window to better understanding of how the resources of this nation have come to be so poorly apportioned and how the resulting structural inequalities have contributed to the spread of leprosy.

Leprosy in Brazil

Why does Brazil have the highest incidence and prevalence of leprosy in the Western Hemisphere and the second highest prevalence of any nation in the world? Leprosy did not exist in the Americas before the arrival of Europeans. In 1500 Portuguese explorer Pedro Cabral captained the first European ship to land on the continent of South America. Although the prevalence of leprosy in Europe had declined dramatically by the fifteenth century in many parts of Europe, it was still a problem in Portugal until the early twentieth century, thus creating one source of the disease in Brazil (Smith 2003). Leprosy was also endemic to the regions of West and Central Africa that were focal to the Portuguese slave trade (Souza-Araújo 1946). In nineteenth-century Rio de Janeiro, white Brazilians attributed the introduction of leprosy to Africans and the African slave trade (Karasch 1987, 162). At least four million Africans were brought to Brazil as slaves (Voeks 1997, 148), and the conditions of slavery contributed to the spread of the disease. Historian Mary Karasch's research on slave life in Rio de Janeiro (1987,146) led her to write that "lack of adequate food, clothing, and housing, in combination with punishment, weakened slaves and prepared them to be finished off by the viruses, bacilli, bacteria, and parasites that flourished in the dense population of urban Rio." On

Brazilian sugar plantations, up to one hundred slaves lived together in a longhouse-type building, the *senzala* (Mattoso 1986, 116), providing the long-term, close contact cited as necessary for leprosy transmission in a population where this disease exists. Since leprosy is not typically fatal except in cases of secondary infection (for example, gangrene might arise from a wound that resulted from nerve damage), statistics on its prevalence are rare. Still, accounts that describe other common conditions among enslaved populations may reveal more about the existence of leprosy. For example, Karasch (1987, 163) notes that blindness was "epidemic" among slave populations in Rio de Janeiro during the nineteenth century. Leprosy may have been the cause of this among some individuals.

After slavery was abolished in Brazil in 1888, many of the former slaves moved to urban areas, where they owned no property and, with little or no income, they built their own homes or shanties. Other Brazilians of mixed or European descent whose ancestors had (or who had themselves) fared badly because of multiple boom-and-bust cycles of the Brazilian economy, general rural poverty, or periodic droughts in the Northeast of Brazil also moved to the cities and became part of favela communities. Urban favelas may have contributed to the spread of leprosy in Brazil, since they tend to concentrate a large number of people in a small area. Also, several people tend to share a small space within each favela home. In a contemporary study conducted in 165 municipalities in the state of Ceará in Brazil, researchers found leprosy to be "associated with a high level of poverty and rapid, unplanned, and uncontrolled urbanization" (Kerr-Pontes et al. 2004, 267). Leprosy is also currently a problem among rural peasants in the Amazon region, where healthcare is less accessible than in the urban areas and where population densities within households is even higher than in the urban megacities. This population density has recently been correlated with leprosy rates in Amazônia in a study by the IBGE (Brazilian Institute of Geography and Statistics) (personal communication, Dr. José Antônio de Nascimento, geographer with IBGE).

Hospitals and isolation facilities specifically for leprosy patients began to appear in Brazil in the mid-1700s. Gerhard Hansen's 1873 discovery that leprosy's causative agent was a bacillus transmissible from person-to-person gave impetus to a new leprosarium era in Brazil and elsewhere (Gussow 1989). In Brazil, there was an increase in both research on and panic about leprosy early in the twentieth century, when the Brazilian government and social elite were attempting to portray Brazil as a progressive industrializing nation. At a conference about leprosy held in the city of Belo Horizonte, Brazil, in 1932, the disease was described as "the most afflicting . . . and the most urgent of all national problems" (Lisboa 1932, 1). Leprosy was considered a sign of backwardness, and its presence was thought to discourage immigration of Europeans, which was considered desirable at the time. The care of leprosy patients was also seen as a drain on national resources.

After the discovery that sulfones were a successful treatment for leprosy, outpatient treatment became a possibility and some leprosarium residents were allowed to leave. However, in the 1960s, perhaps as a result of increased politically repressive policies in Brazil in general during the era of military dictatorship, some people with leprosy who had left the leprosarium were forced to return. I interviewed a physician whose uncle had leprosy; he recalls:

> In Brazil in the sixties . . . there was a new law of segregation passed for leprosy patients to return to the leprosaria. . . . And it was very complicated because I remember I was very small and my uncle—I remember a terrible scene because it was a small city and the people in the North have many preconceptions. So I remember one afternoon they came, opened the door, lassoed him, pulled him by the rope, and forced him into a car. It left me really sad, and truly, I thought right then about entering medicine and within medicine, dermatology.

It was not until the 1970s that forced isolation policies for leprosy patients were changed. There were just over one hundred leprosaria or *hospitais-colônias* (hospital-colonies) established in Brazil, and today, thirty-three of these communities still exist as places where former patients and their families continue to live. I visited one of these colônias, Curupaiti, in the municipality of Jacarepaguá (in the state of Rio de Janeiro), several times during my research, as it also housed an outpatient clinic for leprosy patients as well as the State Institute for

Sanitary Dermatology for Rio de Janeiro. As was the case at Carville in Louisiana, many former patients who were once forced to live in the housing facilities on the grounds of Curupaiti preferred to stay in what had become their home. In contrast to Carville, as I detail elsewhere (White 2003), the families of former patients were allowed to move onto the grounds of Curupaiti, though no new leprosy patients were officially allowed to live there. There has recently been a growth in squatter housing in the area around Curupaiti by relatives of former patients and occasionally even by newly diagnosed patients who hope to take advantage of the resources available to residents of Curupaiti, such as easy access to excellent healthcare. Public awareness of these communities, which in popular belief are still associated with mandatory isolation, contributes to shaping the stigma that surrounds the disease today in Brazil.

In an attempt to reduce stigma associated with the disease, Brazilian leprologists began using the term *hanseníase,* or Hansen's disease, in place of *lepra* (leprosy), and the Brazilian Ministry of Health adopted the term *hanseníase* by 1976 (Oliveira et al. 2003). The NGO I worked with, MORHAN, lobbied for an official name change in the mid-1990s, and in 1995, then-president Fernando Henrique Cardoso signed a law that outlawed use of the term *lepra* in Brazil (*Correio Braziliense* 1995). It is interesting that Brazil took this step. In the United States, there was a strong movement among residents at Carville, in Louisiana, to move away from the terms leprosy and leper in favor of "Hansen's disease" and "Hansen's disease patient" (or "person affected by Hansen's disease"). This movement was successful within the community of Carville. When I was collecting oral histories there, physicians and staff used these terms or an abbreviated form (H.D.). In the international community, however, there has been more resistance to changing the name, in part because "Hansen's disease" does not have the same power to attract charitable donors. The World Health Organization (WHO) continues to use "leprosy," as do organizations such as American Leprosy Missions. I went back and forth several times on whether, in this book, to use the term "leprosy," which perhaps better conveys the history of the disease and its stigma, or the less stigmatizing but also less familiar "Hansen's disease." I primarily use "leprosy," but never "leper" (unless quoting another source or individual). In Brazil, although I do think the term *hanseníase* is helpful in reducing stigma, some of the common stigmatizing ideas and folk models connected with *lepra*, which I discuss further in the next chapter, have come to be associated with the term *hanseníase* in recent years, according to a recent survey (Oliveira et al. 2003).

Today, Brazilians diagnosed with leprosy receive treatment free of charge at public health posts. When I was conducting my research, leprosy treatment was only available at a few referral centers throughout the city of Rio de Janeiro, but an effort is currently underway to decentralize leprosy treatment in Brazil, so that MDT is available to patients at all public health posts (Andrade and Virmond 2004). Though Brazil's efforts to eliminate leprosy and its commitment to advance research on the disease are exemplary in many ways, incidence of leprosy there has decreased only slightly in recent years. To some extent, global leprosy policy has affected the situation in Brazil. I will revisit this issue in the final chapter of the book, but here, I will describe in more detail what life is like for the majority of people affected by leprosy in Rio de Janeiro, since these living conditions provide clues to why this disease continues to be a problem.

The Contemporary Setting

Within the city limits (the municipality) of Rio de Janeiro, there were slightly more than six million residents in 2004 (IBGE 2005), though nearly another six million live in the greater metropolitan area of Rio de Janeiro, which includes several suburbs. According to the 2000 census in Brazil, there were 513 favela communities in greater Rio (Pontes and Schimdt 2001), making up 18.8 percent of the approximately twelve million residents of this area (VivaRio 2005). The favelas constitute a difficult physical environment in which to live. People build their own homes, or *barracos*, out of purchased or collected materials, including paper, cardboard, plastic, tin, wood, brick, or concrete. Whereas early favela homes were commonly made from wattle and daub (mud or clay that holds wood together), today many favela homes are of sturdier construction and are often indistinguishable from those one might see in a lower-middle- or middle-class neighborhood anywhere in Brazil

(Monteiro 2004). Although great care is taken in the construction of many individual homes in the favelas today, this is still a form of what is known as "spontaneous shelter," and so standards for safety in construction are not always met and urban planning has traditionally been minimal.

The standard of living in different favelas varies. Some favelas have been "urbanized," which means that the government, often in collaboration with NGOs and *Associações de Moradores* (Residents' Associations, or community political organizations), pave streets and bring in city services, including electricity, garbage collection, and/or running water. In favelas that were established in the early twentieth century, there are areas where people have been living for several generations, and gradual improvements have been made over the years. Within favelas, there is also a degree of economic and social stratification, visible in quantity of material possessions and in the location and type of one's home. In hillside favelas, for example, there are advantages to having a home toward the top of the hill, primarily because sewage and waste are carried downward to accumulate in the lower parts of the favelas. However, Page (1995) notes that in some favelas, this geographical hierarchy is reversed, as the high-altitude favela homes are less likely to be able to hook up with city services, and the climb for residents is more demanding. It is also harder to carry heavier (and thus, sturdier) building materials, like bricks, to the highest altitudes of the hillside favelas. Wealth differentials within the favela are related to family income, length of time in the city, and the amount of social capital to which people have access. In the favela, valuable social capital would include connections with the Residents' Association, samba schools, a powerful NGO, church leadership, and/or drug trafficking gangs, all of which may be appealed to for funds for home and community improvements.

Individual home improvement is as much or more of a concern of most favela dwellers as it is among middle- and upper-class homeowners. At the base of the favela at the end of the street where I lived in Ipanema, bricks and other building materials were for sale and would be purchased by those interested in putting an addition (usually for other family members, or even for renting) onto their homes. In many favela communities, a number of small businesses flourish; most common are small stores called *biroscas*, where residents can buy basic necessities, and *botequins*, where people can buy beer, *cachaça* (cane liquor), and snacks. On recent (2005 and 2006) visits to the favela of Rocinha, it was clear that this fairly urbanized favela has nearly every type of service available in a neighborhood of the *asfalto* (asphalt, i.e., middle- and upper-class neighborhoods)—clothing stores, pizzerias, internet cafés, video stores, and even a Bob's, the Brazilian fast food equivalent of McDonald's. Favela tourism is a relatively recent source of income for some favela residents (and for tour companies, some favela-based, some not); tourists are brought into the favela to see urban poverty firsthand. Some Zona Sul favelas offer hostel accommodations for tourists; the Favela Hostel, near the beachfront neighborhood of São Conrado, invites tourists to "be a guest in a [secure] slum and feel the amazing experience of being in contact with Brazilian people" (Hostel-Planet.com 2005). These capitalist excursions within the favelas give an appearance of socioeconomic vigor, but favela residents are not always the ones in control of these developments and the profits made (Neuwirth 2004).

Though the exterior environment of the favela neighborhood may contain garbage and sewage, many favela homes are neat and well furnished within. Brazilian store credit plans, which allow people to make multiple installments over several years for even the smallest appliances and furniture items, make it possible for even the poorest Brazilians to accumulate material items within the home over time. On a visit to one favela in 1999 with a MORHAN representative, I remember being impressed with the interior of an office run by an evangelical community leader, complete with computers and fax machines, and with the home of a woman who ran a small school in the favela. Inside the latter, atop the floorboards that seemed like they would collapse under my weight, the room resembled a middle-class home with its cozy furnishings. On multiple visits to a favela NGO with my study-abroad students, I have noticed that the exterior porcelain tiles of some homes resemble those that adorn many of the older Portuguese-style homes in middle- and upper-class neighborhoods in Rio. Though most people do not have the means to lock up their possessions, stealing and other crimes against fellow favela residents are uncommon, in part because there is a degree of vigilante retribution for such crimes against one's neighbor (Goldstein 2003). In my experience, Rio's favelas should not be characterized as "urban hellholes," a label assigned by Joseph Page (1995). However, the idea that people in the favelas are "poor but happy" is another misconception at the opposite extreme of generalization. The reality, I think, is much more complex. The people of the favelas face far more challenges in daily life than middle- and upper-class Brazilians, and they face many obstacles to social mobility, not the least of which are the stereotypes associated with being a *favelado*, the term for a person from the favela that is often used in a derogatory manner by the middle and upper classes.

In the Brazilian media and in the elite imagination, favelados are often constructed as *marginais* (marginals), though as Janice Perlman demonstrated in her book *The Myth of Marginality* (1976), they are neither politically nor economically marginal to Brazilian society. The urban poor are the backbone of the economy of Brazilian megacities. Middle- and upper- class Brazilians are dependent on low-paid domestic workers, serving as nannies and maids, who allow them to increase their household income by freeing both men and women to work outside the home. Men from the favelas also work jobs in the service industry or in construction and other forms of manual labor that are essential for Brazilian society to function.

Stereotypes of favelas as dangerous, crime-ridden, filthy neighborhoods are also common among middle- and upper-class Brazilians. Goldstein (2003, 176) notes that when she told friends from these social strata in Brazil that she was working and living in the favelas, they were "shocked to find that this kind of work was even possible." In Rio, many of my Brazilian and American friends and colleagues lived and/ or worked in favelas, and my husband lived and taught English in the favela of Rocinha in 2006. However, among Brazilians I have met in the United States (many of whom come from the middle- and upper-class segments of Brazilian society), I have also encountered this reaction when I mention that I take American university students to community development projects in different favelas in Rio de Janeiro. Media portrayals of the favelas on the news and in film tend to reinforce stereotypes about the lawlessness and horror of daily life there. For example, the 2002 film *City of God* (*Cidade de Deus*, directed by Fernando Meirelles and Kátia Lund) contains a brilliant portrayal of the development of the drug trade in the public housing complex-turned-favela of the same name. However, by focusing on drug trafficking and those involved in the drug trade, the film reinforces viewers' perceptions of favelas as terrifying and dangerous realms of the "other." Outside of Brazil, perceptions of Rio de Janeiro as a frightening place may have increased because of this film; study-abroad students have mentioned to me that they or their parents had seen this film and were concerned about their safety prior to our trip. After the program, students usually come away with a different perception. As one student wrote about the favela of Rocinha in a post-trip essay, it is "just a neighborhood with stores and adults and kids who were going about their lives." Violence related to drug trafficking and police intervention is indeed a significant problem that affects the lives of many residents. However, community life within the favelas is generally vibrant and alive, and the majority of favela residents are hard-working, friendly, and welcoming individuals.

Favelas are not the only type of community in which the lower socioeconomic class of Rio de Janeiro lives. Public or government housing constitutes another type, although the line that distinguishes the two community types is often blurred, since spontaneous construction is common and unregulated in many public housing areas. In the 1960s and early 1970s, during the military dictatorship in Brazil, many favelas were destroyed and their residents "invited" to relocate to public housing projects. Zona Sul favelas, in particular, were targeted because they were located on prime real estate, where developers were interested in building apartments or hotels that would offer excellent views of the ocean or that would be situated in picturesque locations around Rio. Most of the new government housing projects were built on the periphery of Rio de Janeiro; yet most former favela residents worked in the city or in the Zona Sul. Thus, their displacement made their commute to work more costly and more time-consuming (Perlman 1976). New formal sector job opportunities in these peripheral areas were limited, thus making illegal forms of making a living, particularly drug trafficking, more appealing to some residents. In some public housing communities, an influx of new people into the area has resulted in the development of a shantytown community adjacent to or around the initial housing project.

This was the case with the history of the community of Cidade de Deus. Janice Perlman did fieldwork in Catacumba, a favela once located above the beautiful Lagoa Rodrigo de Freitas, in the Zona Sul. In 1970, this favela was torn down, and many of its residents, along with the residents of several other Zona Sul favelas, were relocated to government housing complexes in the Zona Norte and in relatively isolated and undeveloped land to the west of Rio, in Jacarepaguá. As the film mentioned above also demonstrates, the development of organized crime and drug trafficking had a great deal to do with the distance of this community from previous places of employment. Perlman interviewed former Catacumba residents in Cidade de Deus in 1973 and found that for those who maintained jobs in the Zona Sul, their commute time and expense has increased dramatically. In addition, residents were now required to pay rent, although Cidade de Deus and other housing projects to which people were relocated lacked some of the city services that residents had been promised before the removals (Perlman 1976). Because these areas were relatively unregulated, spontaneous construction sprung up around the housing that was there and, in essence, Cidade de Deus is now considered a favela.

There are also working-class neighborhoods in Rio and its suburbs that are neither favelas nor public housing projects, but the location and quality of people's homes and streets present similar challenges in terms of the urban environment. Residents of the Zona Norte, for example, might as well live on a different planet than those in the Zona Sul. The chic boutiques, jewelry stores, and luxury apartment buildings and hotels of the Zona Sul are absent in the flatland neighborhoods of the Baixada Fluminense in the Zona Norte. Pollution of air, water, and land are more concentrated in these suburban areas to the north of the city where much of Rio's heavy industry can be found. While the favelas represent a kind of lifestyle that does not exist in the United States, since most communities in the United States are equipped with basic sanitation, electricity, and running water, the non-favela lower-middle-class neighborhoods of Rio's suburbs approximate living conditions in North American inner-city housing projects.

Though I did not ask patients I interviewed what type of community they lived in, because I was aware of the stigma that exists surrounding the term *favela*, I did ask where they lived (what part of the city) and asked about some of the difficulties of their daily life and the problems people faced in their community, and this information clued me in on the type of home and community in which they resided. Flooding was a major concern for many of the people I interviewed. In parts of Rio where favelas are built on steep sides of the hills and mountains, flooding often results in landslides that topple and bury homes along with people's possessions, and, when they occur at night, the inhabitants as well. Flooding tends to cause problems for everyone in the favelas, particularly in unpaved areas. In favelas without adequate sanitation, trash and raw sewage fill the ditches that run through the narrow alleyways, and in heavy rains, these waste products may be washed back into people's homes. Sanitation, or lack thereof, was also a primary concern of the patients I interviewed, and many felt, with good reason, that sanitation problems compromised their health. Sylvia Tesh and Eduardo Paes-Machado (2004) have noted that, according to survey data, sanitation is one of the leading concerns among people throughout Brazil.

One patient I interviewed, Renata, thirty-six years old at the time of my interview with her, told me that she had asked a community representative to do something about the ditch that runs in front of her house, but he told her they did not have the resources to fix it. She told me: "Truly, this ditch does me harm [*me prejudica*] because people go throwing garbage in the ditch, and when it rains, my house is the first one to flood. I went to complain. Did it do any good? No." Lorenzo, forty-two, who owned his own house in a favela in Nilópolis, home of the famous Beija Flor samba school, commented: "Look, the greatest difficulty in the community is sanitation. See, where I live . . . if it rains a little, the street fills up. It's a small island and it doesn't support any quantity of water. Where I live, it's lowland. It's a favela. It's all paved; the only problem is when you need to leave the house, because when it rains, the street fills." The open sewers and presence of garbage and trash in the favelas also create problems with a variety of vermin. Fifty-year-old Humberto, a patient, and his wife, Ângela,

who was present during my interview with him, discussed this problem
in their favela community:

ÂNGELA: *Mosquito pra caramba* [Lots of mosquitoes]!

HUMBERTO: Mosquitoes and rats. You're talking about difficulties—the
thing we have most of is rats. The sewer is full. It's terrible.

ÂNGELA: You can't go there without seeing rats—there are lots of rats.

HUMBERTO: . . . I think they should arrange a way to eliminate the
rats from the ditch [valão] or at least reduce the number of them,
because it's really something. It's dangerous. . . . Because I saw a rat
walking near me, I thought it was a cat.

ÂNGELA: Rats bring a lot of illnesses, don't they?

Indeed, many of the most common health problems in the favelas are
borne by rats and mosquitoes. Though malaria and yellow fever, both carried by mosquitoes, are no longer a problem in Rio, dengue fever is quite
common during the rainy season. Leptospirosis, a bacterial infection that
can be transmitted to humans through exposure to animal urine, is common in the favelas primarily because of the large number of rats.

Prevalence of diseases transmitted from person to person is also
high in the favelas and working-class neighborhoods of Rio de Janeiro.
Although there is a high incidence of leprosy in the communities where
the people I interviewed lived, only a few people mentioned this as a
primary disease of concern in their neighborhood. Most interviewees
considered four diseases—TB, HIV, meningitis, and cancer—to be of
greater concern than leprosy. At the same time, having leprosy represented an increased burden to their already difficult lives.

Another serious problem of daily life in the poor communities of
Rio de Janeiro and the number one problem mentioned to me by interviewees is violence. Violence, primarily in the form of shoot-outs that
erupt between drug trafficking gangs within the favelas and between
drug traffickers and police, is a problem in certain areas of the city
where these gangs are more active. Donna Goldstein's book *Laughter out
of Place* (2003) contains an excellent analysis of the development of drug
trafficking in the Rio favelas and its effect on daily life for individual residents. Like Philippe Bourgois (2002), in his detailed work on the lives
of crack dealers in East Harlem, Goldstein notes that young men (and

sometimes women) who become involved in the drug trade often do so because they see it as a step above the opportunities they have open to them in legal employment. The minimum-wage jobs in which their parents or relatives worked obviously did not provide them with opportunities to achieve social mobility, whereas drug trafficking promises a degree of material wealth and the chance, however slight, of getting out of the shantytown or slum. Structural violence, then, in a system where wealth and power is grossly maldistributed, contributes to the development of organized crime and new forms of physical violence.

Two of the patients I interviewed lost members of their immediate family to gun violence. Eugênio, seventy years old, tearfully recounted that his son was shot in the back of the head while sipping coconut milk at a beach kiosk. Xavier, thirty-two, described how his brothers had "gone down the wrong path" and had started robbing buses. They were eventually shot by police. "They didn't even know how to count money; they would do a robbery and then give me the money to hold onto." His brothers were later killed by a quadrilhazinho ("little gang"); Xavier did not make it clear if they were members of the police or of a rival gang, although both are possible.

In addition to direct experience with violence, which some patients reported, there is an undercurrent of violence in Rio de Janeiro and in other Brazilian cities (Linger 1992). Nearly all of the patients I talked with said that violence was a problem in their communities. Every day in the news there are reports of shoot-outs, carjackings, and kidnappings. However, Goldstein (2003) writes that although middle- and upper-class people in Brazilian cities perceive street violence to be an imminent danger, most of those whose lives are actually touched by violence are among the working classes. Gabriela, the wife of a patient I interviewed, had developed extreme anxiety, depression, and panic, simply from living in the city of Rio de Janeiro. Originally from a rural area in the interior of the state, she said, "I was afraid of everything, even going on the bus." Her husband, Wilson, age thirty-six, added, "Because on television, we see the type of violence that's happening here, and we get this way." Gabriela, also in her thirties, said she felt very "desperate," living in such a violent city. "Because there in my land, in the interior, it's so tranquil . . . the moment I retire, I'm moving back there." She suffered from *nervos*, she said, a culture-bound syndrome not unlike "anxiety disorders" or "panic attacks" in contemporary North American biomedical terminology. Scheper-Hughes (1992) correlates the experience of nervos in women in poor communities of Brazil with physical and social stressors, including difficult and dangerous living and working conditions. She sees nervos as a physical expression of structural inequalities and "the violence of everyday life in Brazil," the subtitle of her book *Death without Weeping*.

Corruption among the police, most of whom are low-paid members of the lower-middle class, is a serious problem that contributes to the violence of life in Brazil. Death squads (*esquadrões da morte*) of off-duty policemen, paid by shopkeepers, restaurant owners, and other business people, have been implicated in the murder of street children and homeless adults (Cézar 2004; Penglase 1994). They may also be involved in drug trafficking and can thus facilitate gang warfare through the provision or sale of weapons, or they may be called upon to "settle private grudges" (Page 1995, 242). On one occasion when I was at the office of MORHAN, a volunteer did not come in to the office because there had been a shoot-out between police and drug traffickers in her neighborhood. Someone had been killed, and she felt it was safer to stay indoors. "Better that she doesn't come in today than that she never arrives," one of the other volunteers commented.

On a visit to Rio in 2004, as I walked along the beach in Leblon, I looked up to read a banner carried behind a small plane. Its chilling message was *Bandido bom é bandido morte* (a good criminal is a dead criminal), followed by a request for the readers to vote for a local politician. How is one's status as a bandido established? Do alleged criminals in Brazil receive a fair trial? Under what circumstances were they arrested? These are questions that others have addressed (Bochenek and Delgado 2005), but I will give a brief example of how bandidos are created by the police and the media.

In June 2005, gunfire erupted in Ipanema, on the street below the residence hotel where I was living and where a group of our study-abroad students were staying. Several students converged in my apartment, less concerned for their own safety than interested in getting a balcony view of what was happening, as my apartment faced the main street. The following day, on the news and in the paper, it was reported that a man had been arrested for selling marijuana in the nearby plaza and people in the favela of Cantagalo engaged in a shoot-out with police because they claimed he was just a water deliverer. Two weeks later, we visited an NGO project there. We walked through the favela and down the hill to leave, and I asked our escort, a resident and NGO volunteer, about the incident. He said the man arrested had been one of his students, was not involved in drug trafficking, and was released by the police shortly after being arrested, since there was no evidence against him. The impression left by newspaper reports and by the incident itself, in which, luckily, no one was shot or killed, is that the people of the favelas incite violence, when police are often the instigators of violent acts.

As in the United States, most attempts at dealing with violent crime in Brazil are punitive and do not address the roots of criminal behavior. Brazilian ethics and philosophy professor Renato Janine Ribeiro (2003) notes that even the liberal Partido dos Trabalhadores (PT, or Worker's Party) in Brazil, has moved away from a human rights-based approach in looking at those who commit crimes and toward a rhetoric focused more on law enforcement and "security." Politicians who support harsher sentences for convicted (or even alleged) criminals or who express sentiments like the one mentioned above tend to be more popular among the middle and upper classes than those who propose to address the roots of the problem of crime. The urban poor often receive the blame for crime-related violent acts, though it is this group that is most affected by every aspect of this type of violence.

Getting By

Residents of favelas and other low-income neighborhoods also face the task of making a living in a difficult economic environment. Minimum wage in Brazil is calculated per month rather than per hour. In the late 1990s when I was doing my research, the minimum wage was equivalent to about seventy dollars (U.S.) per month, which calculates to about thirty-two cents an hour for an eight-hour-a-day job. It has since increased and was expected to be raised in April 2008 to R$408.90, about U.S. $229 (Rádio Viva News 2007). Although the minimum wage has been adjusted through the years to accommodate inflation, Mylena Fiori (2004) notes that the amount one can buy on one minimum wage is greatly diminished. For example, in 1959, one minimum wage would cover one thousand city bus rides; in 2004, it paid for 153 rides. A person who needs to take two buses to reach a job location would use up most of their income on transportation alone.

Francisco Neves (2003), citing a study by the IBGE, says that 40 percent of the population of Brazil was living on less than one minimum wage in 2002. Many jobs in Brazil that are not part of the formal economy, within which employers and employees report wages paid or earned to the government, are poorly remunerated. Within the informal economy, although work activity and income may be reported as census data, economic transactions between employer and employee take place "off the books." As mentioned above, a common profession for women in the lower socioeconomic class in Brazil is that of domestic worker. Domestics work (and sometimes live) in the homes of middle- and upper-class families as nannies, cooks, and/or cleaners, and their wages are typically not reported to the government, leaving employers free to pay less than minimum wage for services. Of the twenty-four women I interviewed, nine worked or had once worked as either a domestic servant or a cleaning woman (cleaning in a store or other business or building). Five of these women had been domestic workers in people's homes. Ten of the men I interviewed had at one time had a job in manual labor such as in construction, metallurgy, or woodworking, which required them to lift heavy objects or perform difficult physical tasks. Most of the other work activities reported by the patients I interviewed were also blue-collar jobs that required manual labor of some sort. In addition to being low paying, these occupations are also physically demanding and require repetitive motion that can increase the chances of disability for people with leprosy.

Deus É Dez (God Is Cool): Popular Religion in Rio de Janeiro

Anthropologist and Brazilianist Charles Wagley wrote, in his classic ethnographic description of Brazilian society, *An Introduction to Brazil* (1971), that the Catholic religion, was, along with the Portuguese language, one of the unifying forces in Brazilian culture. At the time he wrote this book, Brazil was over 94 percent Catholic. Over the past several decades, however, evangelical Protestant religions have steadily gained influence in Brazil, particularly among the poor. In 1990, it was estimated that one-sixth of Brazilians were members of a Protestant church (Chestnut 1997). I have observed an increase in the number of storefronts in Rio de Janeiro that have been converted into meeting places for evangelical Protestant churches since my first visit to Rio in 1992. The presence of the evangelical ideology was very noticeable while I was in Brazil and had an influence on popular views of illness.

One of the more powerful of the evangelical churches is the Igreja Universal do Reino de Deus, the Universal Church of the Kingdom of God, or IURD. IURD churches have sprouted up all over Brazil; I often thought of it as a "chain church," with its logo becoming even more prevalent than and as recognizable as McDonald's. Founded in 1977 by Brazilian Edir Macedo, this church has since branched out internationally to over eighty countries (Nascimento 2005). There is a television program in Brazil that is broadcast several hours a day on the Record network. Each day, this program, called *Nosso Tempo* (Our Time), offers a question for the public. They have "reporters" on the street, asking people the question of the day, and they have a phone number for callers. I watched this program occasionally, to try to understand some of the tenets of the Igreja Universal, because I had talked with patients who were members of this church. Although the phone lines are open for anyone to call in, and people can freely express their opinions, the ministers who host the show make the opinions of the Igreja Universal very clear in the course of a program. They do this by hosting interviews in the studio with individuals who have experienced a problem that they believe was solved when they turned to the church. They also have brief prepared videos that suggest the church's answer to the question that has been posed.

I noticed that some of the questions asked on the program have to do with illness. On February 16, 1999, the question was, "Do you believe that undiagnosed illnesses are caused by malignant spirits?" We find out as the program proceeds that the answer of the Igreja Universal is that illnesses that seem to have no medical cure or that are mysterious to doctors may be caused by malignant spirits, and people afflicted by such illnesses should seek help in the church. In particular, they attribute possession or affliction by such spirits to involvement in Afro-Brazilian religions, which are much maligned in many evangelical Protestant churches in Brazil. A woman interviewed in the studio had an undiagnosed illness that cleared up as soon as she became an evangelical. "Jesus is the doctor of doctors," she said, and people who cannot find a good diagnosis "should look for an evangelical church." Footage was shown of a minister giving a sermon in which he talked about "bacteria used by malignant spirits" and said that diseases such as AIDS could be cured through prayer. The Igreja Universal claimed to have cures for continuous headaches, severe back pain, gastritis, bumps and blisters covering the body, and other illnesses that can "fool" (*enganar*) doctors. Evangelical religion in Brazil also tends to appeal to people's distrust for or frustration with biomedicine. Faith healing is offered as a great alternative to medicines and doctors. According to R. Andrew Chesnut (1997, 2), who researched the Pentecostal movement in Belém, illness is one of the key reasons people convert to an evangelical church: "Illness is one of the most common and life-threatening manifestations of poverty in Latin America. . . . Unlike its major religious competitors, Pentecostalism, in all its many denominations, offers the powerful remedy of faith healing."

Though it is losing many of its followers to the charisma of the evangelicals, Catholicism has produced a few of its own dynamic representatives to lure people back or keep people in the Catholic Church. In December, 1998, a huge concert and Mass was held on the beach in Ipanema by Padre Zeca, known as the "surfing priest" (Astor 1998). On the day of the concert, my husband and I saw hundreds of people with the slang expression, *Deus É Dez* (God Is Cool), on their t-shirts. *Deus É Dez* was the theme of the concert and of the CD that was then available in stores and even in the supermarkets of Rio. Gospel-type music sung by Catholic priests has also become popular. Another charismatic Catholic priest in Brazil is Padre Marcelo Rossi, a former gym teacher who leads his congregation in calisthenics and singing: "Rossi regularly draws crowds of 70,000 to the Masses he celebrates four times a week in a former bottle factory on São Paulo's south side. . . . A typical Mass is followed by a 'festinha,' or little party, where Rossi leads the crowd in his 'Aerobics of the Lord'—jumping, singing, and air-boxing" (Astor 1998, 18A). In late 1998 and 1999, when I lived in Brazil, Padre Marcelo's image was ever-present on television. He has since won a Latin Grammy award for one of his CDs in the Best Christian Album category (Astor 2004).

This more charismatic brand of Catholicism has paralleled the decline of liberation theology and of Christian Base Communities (CEBs, *Comunidades de Base*), popular forms of Catholicism that emphasized social and political action over supernatural intervention. According to Chesnut (1997, 173–174), the Roman Catholic Church suppressed these forms of "progressive Catholicism"; in addition, the charismatic renewal in the Catholic Church, with faith healing as one of its main components, seems to have great appeal to many Brazilians, particularly the poor.

Afro-Brazilian religions continue to have a following in Brazil, primarily among the poor but with some middle- and upper-middle-class followers. These syncretic religions are based on a set of deities called *orixás*, whose origin can be traced largely to the Yoruba people of what is today Nigeria (Bastide 1978, 15). West African slaves who were forced to worship in Catholic churches found correspondences to their gods in the Catholic saints. *Candomblé* is generally considered a strictly Catholic—West African mix, whereas variants combine other elements from indigenous South American culture and other religious belief systems (Voeks 1997). *Umbanda* is heavily influenced by Kardecism, or Spiritism, to be discussed below. *Macumba*, though often used as a generic term for "evil magic" in Brazil, has also emerged as a separate religion that blends West African religion, Catholicism, traditional Native American religions, and Spiritism (Page 1995, 365).

On one occasion, a woman in my building got on the elevator with me, carrying several small packages of incense. She made a point to say, "I'm not a *macumbeira*, don't worry. These are just for relaxation. I don't practice *macumba*." The term *macumba* is similar to "voodoo" in the United States, although both terms also designate religions (Voeks 1997). Many nonpractitioners believe that these religions are primarily involved in bringing ill will or harm to others. Much as voodoo (*Vodun*) and *Santería* are portrayed as cults in the United States, focused on spells and sorcery, so also are many Afro-Brazilian religions portrayed in a negative light, particularly among the growing number of evangelical churches in Brazil. In reality, healing and the promotion of well-being are emphasized in Afro-Brazilian religions. Many people who practice Afro-Brazilian religion will say they are Catholic or that they are *Espiritistas* or *Espiritualistas*, Spiritist or Spiritualist, terms that are more ambiguous and also indicate the influence of Kardecism on their religious beliefs. Kardecism (*Kardecismo*), after Alain Kardec, who brought a form of Spiritism to Brazil from France in the nineteenth century, emphasizes the connection between this world and the spiritual or supernatural realm, made possible through possession, séance, and reincarnation. Kardecism was initially popular among whites in Brazil, but the belief system corresponds well with Afro-Brazilian religions, and elements are often combined.

In addition to the religions mentioned above, there are significant numbers of followers of Islam, Judaism, and Buddhism among descendants of different immigrant communities in Brazil (Lesser 1999). The New Age movement also has an influence in Brazil, particularly in terms of alternative-healing choices. Crystals, sold most weekdays on a street corner near the apartment where we lived in Rio, were advertised as having curative powers. Psychic healing, often but not always associated with Umbanda or Spiritism, is also common in Brazil. These types of healing do not necessarily conflict with Brazilians' religious belief systems.

Regardless of religious identification, everyone is exposed in some form or another to powerful beliefs in supernatural phenomena. I noticed that such phenomena linked to various religions are frequently media subjects in Brazil. News programs often feature stories about places or individuals associated with healing miracles. Anthropologist Sidney Greenfield (1999) compared the nature of religion in the United States and Brazil in a discussion of how psychic surgery works among Brazilian subjects. He claims that some Brazilians easily enter an altered state of consciousness because of cultural influences from childhood: "Brazilian culture, in contrast with our own, for example, teaches, reinforces, and rewards fantasy. Children (and adults) who claim to see the Virgin Mary, Saint Francis, some other saint, or other supernatural being not only are not punished or taken to a therapist—as they would be in North America and Western Europe—but are rewarded and held up for praise" (1999, 220). He claims that Brazilians "from just about all geographical regions, classes, and segments of the population" (1999, 220) see and hear about spirit possession, spontaneous or alternative healing, and miracles on a daily basis and thus may be open to suggestion when it comes to these phenomena. However, it is important not to stereotype Brazilians as more "fantasy-prone" than other groups. I think a reasonable generalization is that the consideration of nonempirical phenomena in daily life and in the media is relatively common in Brazil.

For many of the patients I met, religion was an important source of support that provided them with mechanisms for accepting their illness and with hope for the future. The patients were able to find a way to combine the belief that their disease could be cured through supernatural means with an understanding of the necessity of biomedical treatment. I discussed religion with forty of the forty-three patients I interviewed, and of this group, twenty-one were members of Protestant churches, most of them evangelical, including Baptist, Assembly of God, and the IURD; sixteen were Catholic; one followed Spiritism; and three were "unsure." One patient, Ines, forty-two years old, said, "I go to the Baptist Church, but I'm a Catholic," so I counted her in two categories.

However, adherence to one particular faith was fluid for some of the patients with whom I spoke. Vicente, twenty-eight, said that he became more active in his evangelical church after finding out about his disease: "Because even psychologically it helps. Before I wasn't [active]—before discovering this problem. So, when I discovered the problem, I came to church and it helped me a lot, even in the area of rejection, the area of friendship, even in the area of love, in which I wasn't feeling anything. It helped me a lot indeed. Because faith unites."

A few patients were uncertain of where they should go, in terms of religion. I asked Jacira, forty-five years old, what her faith was and if she went to a church. She answered, "No. I think that it's—I'm looking, right? Jesus has so much—we know we need a religion when we get something [a disease] . . . with these problems with the illness. I know I need one. I believe in God. He's always with me. Every moment. But in terms of going to some place, I don't go. [I'm] in search of a religion."

On the other hand, many patients who were members of an evangelical church claimed to be very actively involved in the church and said that the church helped them a great deal in their lives. For many, it seemed to be a central focus of their lives. Humberto, fifty, had been a member of an evangelical church for fifteen years: "To be evangelical is very important in anyone's life because it's an environment of people who are more honest, more true. . . . I don't know how to explain it correctly—we have a different life. I'm good with my life every day. I fight once in a while, I complain. But my life is very marvelous, very good."

Lorenzo, forty-two, in a sermonlike speech that took place during my interview with him, said that his evangelical church, Assembly of God, provided him with a structure for his life and an assurance that his young children would grow up healthy and safe:

> I think about their future. Later they'll be able to get a job. . . .
> [We must] put ourselves in the presence of Lord Jesus, and why?
> The man who is in the presence of Lord Jesus doesn't go to the
> left. He goes forward. What does that mean? He's not going to
> deviate on the wrong path, fall into crime. He's not going to sniff
> cocaine, he won't smoke marijuana. Why? Because he's being
> raised as an evangelical. . . . Many people fall. Why do they fall?
> They didn't read the Word, that which sustains the soul. What
> sustains man, woman, the human being in general is the word
> of God.

Wilson, thirty-six years old and Catholic, said that he enjoys going to church, where they perform a prayer that he says helps him feel "somewhat alleviated" from his problems. Janete, forty-one, a Baptist, commented on how religion helps to structure one's life and be calmer about their illness:

> Those who don't know Christ despair. They think it's the end of
> the world . . . so with a disease like this, they despair. We can
> try to bring the Word, to try to bring comfort to a person. Many
> accept it, others don't. . . . When a person has Christ, he has
> peace and tranquility. . . . As I told you, I would not despair even

if I had a terminal illness—I would just have to pass through it. I wouldn't be the first, nor the last. Why despair? . . . Because for us, Christians, we have eternal life. So for me, the important thing is not life here. The important thing is for Christ to know that I'm saved, understand?

Janete also told me that people at her Baptist church knew she had leprosy, and they were very supportive: "They help [and ask], 'Are you o.k.? How are the medicines going?'"

Public health officials and healthcare workers should not take the presence of religious belief in the daily life of patients for granted. Religion can play a negative role in patients' treatment programs if they are encouraged to abandon medical treatment for leprosy or leprosy reaction. At the same time, religion and religious institutions have the potential to provide both emotional and economic support networks for patients suffering from leprosy. They are a forum through which public health education can and sometimes does take place. For example, a lecture given by healthcare workers from the referral center at a Baptist church, at the request of a patient's (Fernando, age twenty) aunt, resulted in the identification of symptoms in several church members. He told me that "many people came to see it, and many people were directed [to seek help]." MORHAN has recently begun recruiting and training women who are devout members of different religions to identify early leprosy symptoms and to encourage people to seek biomedical treatment. These women also ask patients to bring the medicines back to them so that they may pray over them, thus increasing their efficacy. This *benzedeiras* and *rezedeiras* (women who bless and women who pray) program has already shown signs of success (Artur Custódio de Sousa, personal communication, 2006).

Class, Caste, and Race: Social Immobility in a Dynamic Society

Hanseníase is not a difficulty. It's curable. The problem is this country. What future are [the children] going to have? How can we move forward?

—Gerson, twenty-three, father of two, currently living on a
government pension because of leprosy-related disability

> The most difficult problem, everyone thinks, has to do with the
> [problems] throughout the country. We have to live in a delicate
> situation. Money is short, you know? [We'd like] to reach a level in
> which we could live in a more reasonable situation.
>
> —Ivan, fifty-five years old, currently out of work
> because of leprosy-related disability

The above quotations came from patients in answer to my interview question about what difficulties they faced in their daily lives and in their communities. Rather than discussing local issues, these two men chose to address the broader issue of the problems faced by Brazil as a whole. Both had come to the conclusion that their standard of living was not going to improve through the work they did when they were healthy, much less with the minimal support they received now that they were currently unable to work. In twenty-first-century Brazil, the multiple barriers that make social mobility difficult are still in place.

Two of the major barriers—classism and racism—are legacies of the colonial, and later imperial, era. When we speak or write about race, anthropologists acknowledge that this is an arbitrary category that is defined differently in different contexts and cultures. In Brazil, although racial terms, many of which refer to phenotype, are more flexible than they are in the United States, light skin has traditionally been valued over darker skin. In addition, although there are many poor whites in Brazil, "most African Brazilians today are poor and most of the poor in Brazil are African Brazilians" (Graham 1999, 30). Unlike the United States, Brazil's civil rights movement has only recently begun to achieve some recognition among the general public.

The Brazilian elite have been able to maintain the class stratification system in other ways as well. On the surface, the educational system in Brazil might be seen as the primary vehicle for social mobility, since there are many public universities where higher education is free of charge. However, these universities have limited spots that require good scores on the *vestibular*, a college entrance exam. For the most part, these spots are taken by students who have attended private school or who can afford to get private tutoring for the vestibular. Recent affirmative action programs in some Brazilian universities have made some headway toward addressing this problem, but they are controversial because the quota system they use is based on arbitrary decisions about an applicant's racial category.

A relevant question in relation to the distribution of wealth and resources in Brazil, which, I contend, is directly tied to the high prevalence and incidence of leprosy (and many other curable or manageable infectious diseases), is the following: Can Brazil survive economically without the enormous service class that has existed throughout its history as first a Portuguese colony, then an independent empire, and finally, a republic? I have heard middle-class Brazilians who are left of center on most political issues argue that the Brazilian economy would collapse without the servant class. Goldstein (2003, 75) writes, in reference to the elites' dependence on domestic servants, that many Brazilians discuss the "inability of the economy to absorb the lower-class population in any other productive manner." Any drastic increase in the minimum wage would, many argue, result in economic chaos. All nation-states are, by definition, stratified, or hierarchical, but the degree of social stratification varies around the world today. If a service class is indeed necessary for a nation-state to function and experience economic success for at least some of its population, is it also necessary that this class not have access to decent living conditions that include a living wage, clean/running water, paved streets, and adequate health care?

Goldstein (2003, 37) proposes that the main reason that Brazil has not experienced the kind of revolution that other Latin American nations have seen is that hegemony has been achieved in Brazil, and "where hegemony is realized, coercion is unnecessary." People in the working class do not necessarily aspire to change the system; they would instead prefer to find a better place in the existing class hierarchy. However, some in Brazil who seek social reform have placed their hopes in Luis Ignácio da Silva, popularly known as "Lula," who was elected president of Brazil in 2002 and reelected in 2006. Lula was and is perceived by many to be a champion of the poor, having come from a poor working-class background himself. He was a union leader who also founded the Partido dos Trabalhadores (Workers' Party), under which he ran for president unsuccessfully in 1990, 1994, and 1998, before winning the election in 2002 (Goertzel 2003). Lula has established many programs designed to improve living standards for the lowest-income Brazilians, though the scope of the problem of poverty in Brazil is so wide that anything but drastic changes in the socioeconomic structure of the country will not result in apparent change. Recently, Lula's presidency has been marred by corruption scandals, though he has not been implicated directly in illegal activities. However, contrary to the anticipated rejection of neoliberal economic policies embraced by his predecessor, Fernando Henrique Cardoso, Lula seems to be traveling down a similar path. Neoliberal economic theory posits that international and national corporate investment and free trade will result in greater economic prosperity for all through a kind of trickle-down effect. Privatization of previously government-run agencies, such as social security and segments of the healthcare system, is an example of a neoliberal policy that has been activated in Brazil. To date, neoliberal policies have been shown to widen, rather than shrink, the gap between rich and poor throughout the world.

Throughout this book, I attempt to give examples of the correlation between wealth maldistribution and leprosy because I feel strongly that the nature of poverty in Brazil contributes to the intractable nature of leprosy there as well as in India, Nigeria, Bangladesh, Ethiopia, and other countries where leprosy continues to be a public health problem. My own research is focused more on the level of the individual patient, but I try to situate patients' lives in broader social, political, and economic contexts that illustrate some of the barriers they face in seeking treatment and getting well.

3

Dogs, Ditches, and Disease

Folk and Patient Explanatory Models of Leprosy

During my fieldwork in Rio, I often found myself explaining my research project to Brazilians I knew or met. In the process, I learned how people conceptualized different aspects of this disease. For example, while visiting a public school that served mostly children of the adjacent favela, I told one of the teachers I was studying leprosy, giving him both the terms *hanseníase* and *lepra*. "Oh," he said, "Isn't it true that you can diagnose that by looking someone deep in the eye [*no fundo do olho*]?" This belief does not correspond to the biomedical model of diagnosis, but it falls into the category of what anthropologists have traditionally referred to as "folk models." Folk models, as I use the term, are culturally constructed ways of thinking about, talking about, or categorizing particular phenomenon. Folk models may be passed down from parents or other family members to children; they might also be transmitted through the media or in different forms of popular culture. Folk models are not always uniformly held within a society, and they change through time. With leprosy, folk models can influence, but do not necessarily determine or define, patients' experiences with leprosy treatment. However, because they may form the basis of patients' understandings of leprosy before they are diagnosed with the disease, and because they have the potential to generate fear and stigma, it is important to be aware of what these folk models are.

The term *folk* was first applied by anthropologist Robert Redfield (1930, 1940) to delineate peasant, rural, or "traditional" societies as opposed to urban ones. In his study of a Mexican village called Tepot-zlán, he documented how "folk" and "urban" models of "thinking and acting" could both exist within the same setting but, he said, social class determined which models would be held by different groups. Red-field (1940, 735) wrote that his work "called attention to . . . the process whereby the primitive man becomes a civilized or urbanized man." His implication was that "folk" ways of thinking were less sophisti-cated than the "urban" models. Urban thinking is not necessarily more complex than folk thinking. Today, anthropologists use the term "folk model" somewhat differently. It can be applied to any cognitive model of the world held within a particular group or population, regardless of the level of metropolitan sophistication or education. Folk models might also be referred to as popular, cognitive, or cultural models.

Folk models stem from different sources within cultures. Some beliefs are embedded in ideology and religious belief systems. In India, those with leprosy are often believed to carry the disease into the next life or incarnation, making it a seemingly hopeless situation for them (Carciániga and Herselman 1999). The idea that a person with leprosy (or what has been translated as "leprosy") must have committed a sin or moral transgression and has thus been cursed by God stems in part from Judeo-Christian texts (representing the religious belief system at the time the Torah/Old Testament was written). The concept of feng shui, which has to do with constructing and placing objects in har-mony with nature and with the supernatural realm, is important in an understanding of how the Chinese traditionally conceived of leprosy and other illnesses. For example, an outbreak of leprosy in one village was blamed on the disturbance of the landscape through the digging of a pond in an inauspicious place (Feeny 1964).

Many folk models of leprosy etiology and leprosy treatment may be understood through the principles of sympathetic magic, outlined by Sir James Frazer, author of *The Golden Bough,* a multivolume set of books on religion and culture published in 1922. One of these principles is that "like produces like, or that an effect resembles its cause" (1922, 1); Frazer called this principle the Law of Similarity. In the southern United States, eating collard greens at New Year's is meant to bring about a prosperous year (with more green/money). In some cultures, placing a knife under the bed during childbirth is believed to "cut" the pain. Another important principle of magical or supernatural thinking that exists cross-culturally is the Law of Contagion, in which "things which have once been in contact with each other continue to act on each other at a distance after the physical contact has been severed" (1922, 1). For example, in one contemporary folk discourse, people who receive a donated organ inherit some of the memories and feelings of the organ donor.

There are numerous examples of how the principles of sympathetic magic apply to folk models of leprosy. In the Torah/Old Testament, it is said that Pharaoh, King of Egypt, had leprosy and was told, by Egyptian "magicians" or healers, to bathe in the blood of Israelite children. Whether or not such a cure was ever attempted, the idea of blood as a cure for leprosy represents the principle of the Law of Similarity, since "Pharaoh became ill with an illness manifested in wounds on the skin, from which liquid or blood oozes. Since the illness is manifested in blood, the cure is by blood" (Bar-Ilan 2002, 394). Medical theory in South Asia and China once held that leprosy came from eating fish, in part because fish frequently had lesions themselves, and thus, like produces like. Since nerve damage from leprosy makes patients more susceptible to injury and subsequent infection, leprosy often results in gangrene, or "rotten" flesh. In the early twentieth century, a physician who published in the medical journal *The Lancet* proposed "'the rotten meat of aquatic animals' as the causative organism" (Feeny 1964, 45). A nineteenth-century physician (Sandreczki 1889, cited in Tebb 1893, n.p.) referred to the consumption of putrid food as causing leprosy, including "the oil and fat (used for food), rancid, or salted beyond measure; olives and cheese in a state of decomposition; meat rotten, or coming from animals diseased, or worse still." Several of the folk models of leprosy in Brazil can be interpreted through religious ideology or through the laws of sympathetic magic, as will be demonstrated below.

Although folk models are usually contrasted or compared with empirical or scientific models of the world, scientific models may also be understood as "folk models," because they are also the product of a way of thinking about and categorizing the world within a particular cultural and historical framework. Though scientific truths may exist—on

Earth, we can count on a ball falling when dropped, for example—many scientific models, though they may be based on observation and hypothesis testing, change through time and are subject to the influence of political, social, economic, and other forces. For example, the science on nutrition has shifted dramatically over time. For example, when I was growing up in the 1970s, we learned that a balance of the "four food groups" (milk products, meat, breads, and fruits/vegetables) constituted a healthy diet. In 1992 the Food and Drug Administration introduced the Food Pyramid; in this model, the majority of daily calories should come from carbohydrates. A more complex Food Pyramid was designed by the FDA in 2005 to take into account new findings related to nutrition and obesity control. Although science is the purported basis of the different manifestations of nutritional models promoted by the U.S. government, politics is also involved in how these models are shaped. Several agricultural and food-related business interests have lobbying power that influences the construction of the pyramid by FDA officials (Harvard School of Public Health 2005). In this and in many examples of what is presented as pure scientific knowledge, it is difficult to separate "facts" that come out of scientific inquiry from the context in which this information is gathered, since scientific research is often funded by outside sources. Scientists, too, are products of their society and bring with them biases that may affect their approach to research and their interpretation of data.

During my research in Brazil, I was able to determine what some of the contemporary folk models of leprosy were from formal and informal interviews with patients, healthcare workers, and volunteers. Casual conversations with Brazilian friends or acquaintances who were not directly affected by the disease were useful in helping me identify some of these models. Self-help group meetings and educational sessions I attended that were led by social workers or volunteers also elicited folk models of leprosy. Finally, at the favela school I periodically visited, I gave four short talks about leprosy symptoms and treatment to parents whose children attended the school. Before I began these talks, I asked people if they had heard of "lepra," and what, if any, ideas they had about it. The responses were useful in discovering different folk models of leprosy in Rio and the key ideas and terms used in these models.

I used qualitative methods to collect the folk models I describe here, and I am not able to say with any degree of certainty that a certain percentage of the Brazilian population is aware of a particular model of leprosy. However, I attempted to verify each folk model I heard by discussing them with people in different contexts and looking for sources in the academic literature that might corroborate the information I collected. For example, one of the first folk models about leprosy that I heard in Brazil was that it "comes from" dogs. After hearing this rather unique folk model, which will be discussed in more depth below, I spoke with several healthcare workers and MORHAN volunteers, who believed that indeed this was one of the more common folk models of leprosy etiology in Brazil. Interviews I conducted with patients confirmed that this model exists. In addition, a few Brazilian social scientists (Claro 1995; Oliveira et al. 2003) have mentioned the existence of this folk model. These multiple forms of cross-checking information help to verify qualitative information collected from individuals.

Folk Models versus Patient Explanatory Models

People affected by leprosy in Brazil are often familiar with the folk models associated with the disease. However, understanding what these folk models are does not give us a clear picture of how patients conceptualize this disease. Patient understanding of leprosy is shaped or transformed by their personal experience with this illness. When we discuss patients' cognitive models of disease, the term explanatory model, now commonly referred to as "EM" in public health and medical anthropological discourse, may be more useful. For Arthur Kleinman (1980), who coined the term, an explanatory model of illness is just that—a model for explaining, thinking about, and conceptualizing all aspects of that illness. Explanatory models that people subscribe to may affect the decisions they make about health care.

I quickly noticed that patients' explanatory models did not mirror the Brazilian folk models of the disease. Patient explanatory models often combined elements of folk models and medical models of the disease. They came into the clinic with a set of beliefs about Hansen's disease or leprosy and then were exposed, through conversations with doctors, nurses, social workers, psychologists, and other healthcare professionals to one or possibly multiple versions of the biomedical model of their illness. In addition, patients had their own personal experiences with the disease. They compared their experiences with what they have heard from friends, relatives, co-workers, and medical personnel, and using this information, they constructed personalized explanatory models of the disease. Several patients' explanatory models were also influenced by the structural inequalities that affected their daily lives, particularly in terms of how they perceived their living conditions to have contributed to or caused their illness. Some patients were not convinced by or did not completely understand the medical explanations. Others were eager to accept the biomedical version of the disease, though in some cases they found that their subsequent experiences contradicted the medical information they were given about leprosy upon diagnosis. Patient models, then, were constantly shifting to match the patient's experience of disease and treatment at any particular time.

Understandings of *Lepra* versus *Hanseníase*

Before discussing patient explanatory models, I should make it clear what terminology was being used with patients and what illness patients understood themselves to have. As mentioned in chapter 2, *hanseníase,* or sometimes just "hansen" is a term that is now regularly used by doctors and the media to refer to the disease caused by *Mycobacterium leprae.* Awareness of the term *hanseníase* is growing in Brazil as it is used in many public health campaigns on television; "*Hanseníase Tem Cura*" (Hansen's Disease Is Curable) can be seen on posters in health posts and on public transportation throughout Rio. Of the forty-three patients I interviewed, twenty said they had heard the term before (either because they had seen a poster about the disease, seen a commercial about it on television, or knew someone who had it). The term *lepra*, however, has not disappeared from the popular imagination. The use of the term *hanseníase* has created, for some, an idea that hanseníase and lepra are two separate diseases. In a documentary made in the early 1990s, people polled on the streets of Rio tended to describe *hanseníase* as a curable skin disease and *lepra* as a highly contagious disease sent as a punishment from God (Thielen and Coimbra 1992). More recently, however, it seems that *hanseníase* has come to be synonymous with *lepra* for many people. A recent, extensive survey, conducted by Maria Leide Wand-del—Rey de Oliveira et al. (2003) in Rio de Janeiro demonstrated that traditional, often stigmatizing, concepts associated with *lepra* have begun to be associated with *hanseníase*.

Among the people I interviewed, there was a wide range of understanding and interpretation of these two terms. One of my interview questions was, "Had you heard the word *lepra* before [your diagnosis]?" Nearly all patients were familiar with the term. Many knew it was a synonym for *hanseníase*. A few patients believed that *lepra* is what they would get if they did not comply with the treatment program for *hanseníase*. Some patients, however, did not seem to know why I was asking the question—of course they had heard of lepra, but that was not the disease they had. Other social scientists working in Brazil have found similar results in patient perception of terminology. In Marcos Queiroz and Maria Puntel's study of leprosy patients in Campinas (São Paulo state), nearly half of their interviewees "did not consider hanseníase and lepra to be the same or they considered both as very different stages of the same disease, in which lepra is the much more serious manifestation" (Queiroz and Puntel 1997, 93).

Seven patients I interviewed knew they had *hanseníase* but clearly did not associate this term with *lepra*. I was unsure if it was my role to let these patients know that the terms were synonomous, and I felt that talking about *lepra* might create fear where it did not previously exist. I asked Wilson, thirty-six, if he had heard the word *lepra* before. He responded, "That I've heard. Right, with that there is stigma. There's a guy here who's being treated for this business of lepra." He did not know about the connection between the terms nor that everyone at this particular clinic was being treated for leprosy. Heloísa, twenty-three, also seemed confused by my question about her understanding of the term *lepra*, "because this here is not lepra, right?" she said. There are patients who complete their entire treatment program without associating their illness with "leprosy" or *lepra*, since some healthcare workers deliberately avoid reference to *lepra* when speaking to patients. One social worker told me that she never uses the word *lepra* unless the patients themselves bring it up. Otherwise she works only with the term *hanseníase*. She believed that if patients do not know they have lepra, there will be less anxiety and self-stigmatization.

In the patients I interviewed who were unaware of the connection between their illness and lepra, I observed less of a perceived stigma about what they had, although this is difficult to determine from a small sample. Still, I believe physicians should consider using both terms when giving a diagnosis. Patients who are unaware of a connection may not hesitate to tell others they are in treatment for hanseníase; this may generate stigma for the individual if friends or employees know this is leprosy. Knowledge of the synonymous use of *lepra* and *hanseníase* gives patients a chance to make a more informed choice about disclosing their illness. Another factor involved is the fact that *hanseníase* is a somewhat strange word in Brazilian Portuguese, as the base of the word is the Norwegian name Hansen. Neither its spelling nor its pronunciation is common in Brazil. One patient I met had Brazilianized the spelling of the word; a friend had told him to go into the clinic for hanseníase, and he had written on a piece of paper "Rançeníase" (a phonetic spelling in Brazilian Portuguese). The foreign-sounding name may frighten patients who have never heard of the disease. Meanwhile, the term *lepra*, although associated with stigma, is at least understood by patients. Lenita Claro (1995, 50) notes that many of the patients she interviewed had trouble remembering the word *hanseníase*, and the majority "had trouble pronouncing it," primarily because it was an unfamiliar term.

Patients I interviewed who did know about the Hansen's disease–leprosy connection said that they knew that if untreated, they could become disabled or disfigured, just like patients in the leprosaria. Sônia, forty-four, whose narrative is featured in chapter 6, talked about her feelings concerning the two terms:

C.W.: Had you heard the word before?
SÔNIA: Oh, yes. Not "hansen." "Lepra."
C.W.: And were you afraid of this?

SÔNIA: Very much. Well, the first impact. Lepra. Because people told me you have to stay far from your family, you fall to pieces [*cai em pedaços*]. . . . If you go to a colony, you see mutilated people. For me, it's not a legend. It's reality. . . . Hanseníase—only the name has changed. . . . It's the same disease. If you get treatment, [you can be all right], but it's the same thing. . . . It is lepra. I'm an evangelical, so I was in the colony [a former leprosarium, visiting with her church]. People there would look at me, at my appearance and say, "You don't have this disease." Then I'd say, "I had it. I had it and I went through treatment. I'm always in reaction." Then they say, "No, you didn't have it. You have eyebrows, I don't. I have a mutilated nose, you don't." People have those things, right? You know that if you don't get treatment, you're going to be like that.

Some patients who recognized the connection between the two terms felt that *hanseníase* is a euphemism used by doctors to talk about leprosy or to hide the truth from patients. Patrícia, twenty-three, commented that changing the name did not change the disease:

I think that it's all just names—for example, "radio." The name could change but it continues to be the same thing. Of course hanseníase is a prettier word than lepra. But I think it doesn't matter. . . . It's just a word. If I say, "I have hanseníase," it's the same thing as if I say, "I have lepra." The same thing.

Still, Patrícia says she tells very few people about her illness, but with people she trusts, she usually says she has lepra, because "there are people who, if I say, 'I have hanseníase,' they don't know it. If I say 'lepra,' they know."

In writing about popular conceptions or folk models of leprosy in Brazil below, for the most part I am referring to folk models of lepra, not hanseníase, since many people were unfamiliar with the latter term and did not have folk models associated with this word. However, explanatory models for patients I met were all of hanseníase, since this is the term they were given in the health post. As is clear below, however, their conceptions of hanseníase were often intertwined with the popular folk models about lepra.

Uma Doença Que Pega (A Disease You Can Catch): Models of Leprosy Transmission

In analyzing folk models and patient explanatory models of an illness, it is important to look at all aspects of how that illness might be understood. This includes an investigation into how people understand a disease's or illness's etiology, transmission, symptoms, complications, treatment, and cure. George Foster, one of the pioneers of medical anthropology as a distinct subfield, divided "non-Western" etiological belief systems into two major categories—naturalistic and personalistic. Personalistic systems attribute illness to the "active, purposive intervention of an agent" (Foster 1976, 775), such as a supernatural being or a human possessing supernatural powers. In naturalistic systems, illness is believed to come from "such natural forces and conditions as cold, heat, winds, dampness, and above all, by an upset in the balance of the basic body elements" (1976, 775). In many cultures, the body is understood as being composed of different "humors." Humors are tangible (like blood, phlegm, and bile in early European medical thought) or intangible (like yin and yang in traditional Chinese medicine) substances that, if not in balance, can cause illness.

Within most contemporary cultures, there is a pluralism of etiological beliefs about illness. Nearly all societies around the world have been exposed to some aspect of biomedical theory, which does not clearly posit either naturalistic or personalistic causes for illnesses. In Brazilian society, popular understandings of illness, health, and the body merge elements of traditional European, African, indigenous South American, and many other traditions with scientific or biomedical models. The numerous cognitive models of leprosy etiology that I collected in Rio de Janeiro do not, as a group, fit neatly into one or the other system, though some individual models might be characterized as personalistic or naturalistic.

Although the most commonly cited mode of transmission from a biomedical perspective is person-to-person contact, there is still a degree of doubt related to other environments in which leprosy bacilli might reside and how it might be transmitted to humans. On the World Health Organization's (WHO) Web site, for example, there is the following statement about leprosy transmission:

The exact mechanism of transmission of leprosy is not known. At least until recently, the most widely held belief was that the disease was transmitted by contact between cases of leprosy and healthy persons. More recently the possibility of transmission by the respiratory route is gaining ground. There are also other possibilities such as transmission through insects which cannot be completely ruled out. (WHO 2005c)

Given the uncertainty that exists in the scientific model, we might think twice before dismissing patient explanatory models of contagion, many of which are based on an understanding of germ theory. For example, at Carville in Louisiana, one former resident and patient was convinced he acquired leprosy through exposure to the bacillus in the soil in which armadillos (known to carry *Mycobacterium leprae*) regularly rooted; as the son of migrant laborers in Texas, he worked in agricultural fields as a child. Although there is no scientific evidence for this form of contamination, several mycobacteria are known to reside in soil, so from a scientific perspective, it is a reasonable hypothesis on his part.

The first seemingly uniquely Brazilian folk model of leprosy etiology that I learned while doing my research was that leprosy is carried by dogs. This belief may originate in part from a terminological phenomenon with origins in the translation of the Hebrew word *tzaareth* in the Bible to "lepra." This term and its derivatives in other languages (such as "leprosy" in English or "lèpre" in French) have been used in historical texts to describe several different diseases, including elephantiasis, smallpox, bubonic plague, mange, lupus vulgaris, syphilis, acne, ringworm, psoriasis, pellagra, vitiligo, leishmaniasis, eczema, syringomyelia, facial paralysis, and others (Ortner and Putschar 1985, 178).

After I heard the idea that leprosy is carried by dogs, I noticed in my pocket Portuguese-English dictionary that the word *lepra* is translated as both 'leprosy' and 'dog mange' (Bárbara et al. 1989). If *lepra* is also mange (a form of scabies) in Portuguese, then it is not a misconception to say that it "comes from dogs." Many people then confound this lepra with the disease in humans that is caused by *M. leprae*, though some are aware of different types of lepra. For example, when I asked a street vendor of medicinal plants if he had any treatments for lepra, he asked me if it was leprosy of "animals or humans?" Though I answered "humans," there was no guarantee that we were talking about the same disease, since "human" lepra might refer to numerous problems with the skin. Part of the justification of officially changing the name of leprosy to *hanseníase* in Brazil was the association of the word *lepra* with a variety of skin ailments.

The association of dogs and leprosy may be reinforced by the common depiction of dogs licking the wounds of the Catholic saints most closely linked with the disease, Saint Lazarus (São Lázaro) and Saint Roch (São Roque). Connection with impurity is another possible explanation of why dogs are also associated with leprosy. Dogs are considered unclean animals in Muslim societies; while the Koran does not specifically say that dogs are "impure," some of the *hadiths*, or stories of various pronouncements of the prophet Mohammed, contain comments about dogs that indicate their spiritual uncleanliness. Dogs were not supposed to be let into the domestic space of the house; utensils that have been licked by dogs had to be cleaned "seven times" with earth and water; if a dog passed in front of a person who is praying, the prayers were "annulled" (Muslim Student Association–University of Southern California 2002). There is a history of Islamic influence in Portugal and West Africa, both of which made significant contributions to Brazilian culture.

In interviews with volunteers at MORHAN, I asked where they thought this belief originated. They told me that since dogs with mange (*lepra*) often exhibit bad skin problems and have difficulties with their paws, people think that dogs have leprosy. One woman at a self-help group meeting told me she had named her dog "leprinha" (little leper) since it always had open sores. Several parents I spoke with at the favela school meetings I attended also expressed the belief that lepra comes from dogs.

Although the folk model associating dogs and leprosy is common in Brazil, very few of the patients I interviewed thought that contact with dogs was the source of their illness. Their exposure to the biomedical model and/or their personal experiences had led them to believe otherwise. Xavier, thirty-two, considered this possibility along with many other etiological models he entertained. He said that he may have acquired leprosy because his mother allowed her dog to come in the house. Though dogs are highly pampered indoor animals in middle- and upper-class households, they are typically considered outdoor animals in low-income communities. Laura, who was in her forties at the time of my interview with her and had come to Rio from the Northeast of Brazil, said that the belief that lepra comes from dogs is very common in that part of the country. She told me that her husband, also from the Northeast, threatened to leave her because she had "dog leprosy" (*lepra do cachorro*), which he perceived as being highly contagious. Physicians at the clinic where she was being treated were able to convince him that her disease was neither incurable nor contagious once she had begun treatment and that it did not come from dogs. Bringing animals indoors may be seen as a means of spreading animal diseases to humans.

The idea that leprosy can be contracted through eating certain foods, such as fish or pork, is fairly common in Brazil. Sinésio Talhari and René Neves (1997, 2) mention fish and pork as foods that are popularly believed, in the Amazon, to carry leprosy. Although there are no dietary taboos associated with or cultural models of fish or pigs as unclean animals in Brazil, as mentioned earlier in this chapter, beliefs linking particular foods and leprosy were common in Europe, Asia, and Africa as well as in medical theory, and may have diffused to Brazil. A social worker at Curupaiti told me that it is a fairly common belief in Rio that one can get leprosy from eating pork, and a person asked about this in an educational meeting at an outpatient clinic where both leprosy and general dermatology patients were being treated. Among patients I interviewed, only one person mentioned food-borne contamination as a possible source of leprosy. Xavier, thirty-two, told me:

> I worked in Barra da Tijuca [neighborhood south of Rio de Janeiro] for three years, and there was this [swampy area] full of fish. So I went there, fished a lot, and brought them home. No one wanted to eat them, so I ate them all.

I did not ask him at the time if the connection between eating fish and getting leprosy was based on an association of fish and leprosy or a more general association of environmental contamination with disease, since many water sources in Rio de Janeiro are heavily polluted.

Germ theory is now part of the popular imagination in much of the world. Urban Brazilians are familiar with this concept, and many explanatory models of contagion described to me by patients I interviewed were related to the idea of "catching" or "picking up" (*pegando*) diseases from sources that they knew were the vectors of other bacterial or viral agents. Beth, nineteen, associated her disease with time spent playing in a polluted river when she was younger:

> I don't think anyone in my family had it. But where I lived . . . near the river—the river is very rotten [*podre*], right? So, I used to go into the river to retrieve a ball. I was a kid, twelve, thirteen years old, and shortly after, I came down with this disease. Because he [a doctor] said that it comes from dirt [*sujeira*] and then from the family. And I lived near the river. I had a lot of contact [with the river]. . . . I was living there in Manguinhos [a favela]. I got it there. Now I'm living in my husband's house. There it's decent. There's no river, nothing like that.

Some physicians tell patients that their living conditions may contribute to their having contracted leprosy, which is true in the more abstract sense of lowering immunity and increasing susceptibility. Patients sometimes take that to mean that the bacilli themselves reside in garbage, dirty water, or animals. As noted above, it is difficult to dispute the possibility that these are vectors of transmission when there is still some uncertainty in the biomedical model of etiology.

The wind (*o vento*) was mentioned by a few patients as a possible vector of transmission. In many naturalistic etiological systems, the wind might be a force that upsets humoral balances and causes illness. However, since doctors tell patients that leprosy is transmitted "through the air," patients may connect this to "the wind." Although he was familiar with the folk model in which leprosy came from the wind, Manoel, thirty, was skeptical and reasoned that everyone would have leprosy if that were true.

The beach is another ecologically contaminated location that some patients linked to their disease. Regina, thirty-four, thought she got leprosy at the beach: "I used to go to the beach a lot. The beach is not very clean. There are a lot of animals on the beach. I must have caught it there." Regina's model also incorporates the folk belief that leprosy comes from animals. At the beach, Brazilians also wear very little clothing and thus a large proportion of their skin's surface is exposed, which may lead to the idea of increased vulnerability to skin contamination.

Another folk model of contagion in Brazil that has been reported in the literature is that leprosy derives from "burned blood." Talhari and Neves have written that some Brazilians "believe that the blood is 'burned' after a person drinks liquor (*aguardente*) and takes certain medicines—'burned blood' (*sangue queimado*) is a synonym of skin disease, and this is a synonym of MH (Morbus Hansen), principally in the North of Brazil" (Talhari and Neves 1997, 2). Xavier, thirty-two, told me that he overheard a relative telling someone he (Xavier) had "bad blood" (*sangue ruim*) because of leprosy or perhaps as a description of his condition, though he considered this as coming from *gente mal-informado* (people who are ill-informed). Interestingly, Ron Barrett (2005) cites the idea of "bad blood" (and subsequent bloodletting as a treatment) as an explanatory model associated with leprosy among some patients in India. Barrett sees this explanation as a way for patients to justify self-mutilation, which, for leprosy patients who practice begging, translates to greater economic revenue, but the belief may originate in both Brazil and India from humoral understandings of the body.

Patients at the clinic where I spent most of my time received a fairly thorough orientation about leprosy when they were diagnosed; thus many repeat the biomedical explanation that leprosy comes from contact with other people, through their respiration. This explanation leads many patients to conclude that leprosy is easily transmissible from one person to another, which corresponds with popular folk models of leprosy as a highly contagious disease. Patients who had never, to their knowledge, had "intimate and prolonged contact" (in medical literature, an oft-cited condition for transmission) with anyone with leprosy can only theorize that they may have come into contact with someone on the street or in a bus or on the job who had the disease. Humberto, fifty, speculated:

> I don't know where I got this. Maybe from someone else's cloth-
> ing—I don't know if you can get it that way. It's not easy to

understand. I'm a driver, a private [car] driver for a long time in the Zona Sul of Rio. There they have a lot of these things, we don't even know. So many times I've brought these types of medications, skin creams, to people. I don't know if these people had this disease and that I could have taken someone's arm [helping them from the car]. And I had the first [lesion] here on my arm. . . . I don't know, but I think [that could be how I got it].

Humberto made a direct connection between having touched someone and later noticing the appearance of a lesion in that area of his body.

Some patients believe they acquired their disease during a visit to a hospital or, in particular, to a location where leprosy patients were treated. Zé, fifty-five, said he spent some time at the former leprosarium (or *hospital-colônia*) of Curupaiti, visiting his ex-wife's aunt: "There they have this disease. And I like to stroll around, walk, these types of things, visit with people—I think I caught it there. It's the only place I know [where I could have been exposed]—in Curupaiti in Jacarepaguá." At the outpatient clinic on the grounds of the former leprosarium where I attended educational meetings for patients, those who did not have leprosy but came in for dermatological problems expressed their fears about catching leprosy while they were there. From a biomedical view, as one social worker explained during one of these meetings, the odds of catching leprosy there are actually much lower than catching it on the bus or in certain neighborhoods, because the residents were cured and thus no longer transmitting the disease. Still, it is easier to conceptualize contracting leprosy from a leprosarium patient, some of whom have obvious deformities related to the disease, than from a neighbor who has no apparent symptoms.

Patients who had known or seen someone who had leprosy sometimes attributed their disease to contact with these people. Fernando, twenty years old, proposed:

I live in Belford Roxo; I was living in Roxa Miranda [both neighborhoods in the Baixada Fluminense lowlands area north of Rio]. And in Roxa Miranda—I had a friend who had spots—he was covered with spots. Truly covered. I think it was hanseníase. I think I got it from him. Five years ago I got it, in '93.

For Fernando, the visible signs of illness that his friend exhibited were indicators of a contagious disease. From a biomedical perspective, however, patients may exhibit the signs he described after beginning treatment for leprosy, when they are no longer at risk of transmitting the disease to others.

The idea of "prolonged and intimate contact" or "intimate relations" leads some patients to believe that leprosy is sexually transmitted. Two patients, both men, mentioned having possibly acquired leprosy through sexual relations with women. In Portuguese, the word "relations" (relações) often implies sexual intercourse, and the word "intimate" (íntimo) also suggests this type of relationship. Walter, twenty-eight, told me the doctors said that one could get leprosy from an "intimate relationship." "If it was like this," he said, "through 'relations,' it could be this girl. This girl died . . . she was my girlfriend. She died, and it's hard to say whether it was from this [leprosy] or something else." Most likely, his girlfriend died from another disease. Although it is possible to acquire leprosy from a person one spends a great deal of time with, the biomedical view is that it is not transmitted through intercourse, although this was commonly believed by doctors in the Middle Ages (Brody 1974). Among the many theories espoused by Xavier, thirty-two, about the etiology of his illness, he suspected it could have been "from women," he said, "because I worked security for baile funk [dance and music parties that originated in the favelas], [and] every week I'd go out with a different woman."

Religion was involved in the etiological models of a few patients I interviewed. Many Catholic, Protestant, and Afro-Brazilian religious explanations of disease origin are personalistic in nature. Within Candomblé and other Afro-Brazilian religions, disease is sometimes viewed as the result of a curse or feitiço (spell) placed upon the patient by another party. Another possibility is that the patient did not pay proper tribute to a particular orixá. In evangelical churches, unexplained or undiagnosed illnesses are often said to be a result of possession by a demon or the Devil. People "allow" demons into their life by not being vigilant enough. Since leprosy has been constructed as a punishment or curse from God in the Judeo-Christian tradition, this belief also shows up in Protestant and Catholic believers in Brazil. According to Manoel, "if a person has to go through this, I think it's written. Because people have to suffer . . . because if you don't suffer, life has no value." Jacira, forty-five, was unsure about how she got the disease, but her grown children offered suggestions:

> My son, who was twenty-two at the time—he was in the Church. He is a Cristão. I was in bed with these pains, these pains. So my son said this: "Mom, go to church. You have the Devil in your body." I said, "Oh, my son!" I was so afraid when he said that. I said, "Son, don't talk that way. . . . God is always with me. Look at your mother. God doesn't leave me alone. . . ." Then, my daughter was telling me . . . that some were saying that it was a feitiço. Each one [of the children] getting involved in my life!

Jacira ultimately rejected both children's models of how she got leprosy, although she attempted a cure through her daughter's religion (described later in this chapter).

Social workers and physicians I spoke with confirmed many of the etiological theories I elicited from interviews as common beliefs about leprosy contagion. Patients interviewed by Claro (1995) in Rio mentioned the following as possible sources of leprosy etiology: dogs and other animals, eating pork, the wind, open sewers and other environmental pollutants, and supernatural forces such as karma and tests from God (Claro 1995). Queiroz and Puntel (1997) say that patients they interviewed in Campinas, São Paulo, talked about bad habits (smoking, drinking), lack of hygiene, factors related to standard of living (including poor diet, adverse conditions of work, pollution, and lack of access to medical services), problems in patients' personal lives, the evil eye, and macumba as sources of leprosy.

Understanding Symptoms

In Brazil and many other parts of the world, secondary effects of leprosy are often confused with symptoms. In other words, most people associate leprosy with advanced stages of the multibacillary form of the disease, rather than its early symptoms. Leprosy is not popularly thought of as a disease that shows itself initially as a small depigmented mark on the skin, but as a disease in which individuals are horribly deformed. As will be discussed in the next chapter, many physicians in Brazil do not recognize leprosy until it has already done great damage to the individual. Several Brazilian models about leprosy match those I had learned growing up in the United States: that leprosy is highly contagious and causes your flesh to rot and fingers and toes (or arms and legs) to fall off; that people with leprosy live in "colonies" and are isolated from the rest of society; and that leprosy patients are bandaged from head to toe to cover their open wounds. These folk models are based on a mixture of representations of leprosy in film and television and to some extent on historical realities of leprosy. It is important to reiterate that rotting flesh and loss of digits or limbs are not symptoms of leprosy, though complications from secondary infections can cause severe disability. In Brazil, the phrase "*cai em pedaços*" (fall to pieces) commonly accompanies any discussion of lepra. An all-over body itch is associated with lepra in Brazil as well. Itching is not a sign of leprosy, though some patients experience itchy skin at one point or another as a medication side effect or because of dry skin. Most likely, this folk model derives from use of the term *lepra* to refer to mange or scabies, which does produce itchiness.

The image that Brazilians have of the disease may be influenced by a famous countryman who had leprosy. He was an eighteenth-century baroque sculptor from the state of Minas Gerais whose mother had been a slave. Born Antônio Francisco Lisboa, he was better known as Aleijadinho (Little Cripple). *Aleijado* (crippled) is considered a derogatory term today in Portuguese, as in English, but one that is still used to refer to him. Because of his disease, he could no longer use his hands after age thirty, but he continued to sculpt by strapping his tools to his arms (Draffen et al. 1996; Page 1995). Although he is a cultural icon in Brazil, his name and the disease associated with it contribute to the image of leprosy as a disfiguring and incurable disease.

The patients I interviewed who were in treatment for leprosy, if they were in fact aware that their illness was lepra, had learned from healthcare workers that these models were, for the most part, not the reality for them. Before diagnosis, however, very few patients took their symptoms seriously in the initial stages of their disease because they did not associate depigmented spots, numbness, or nerve damage with leprosy. Sixteen patients of the forty-three I interviewed did not go to a physician at the onset of symptoms, thus delaying treatment for months or even years. Patients frequently mistook minor symptoms for a fungus, age or liver spot, or a minor problem that they might have acquired swimming in the ocean or from spending time in the sun. Afonso, age fifty-one, said that he noticed a spot, and his wife urged him to go to the doctor, but he did not connect the spot to a problem. "I didn't feel anything," he said. Denise, twenty-seven, also said she did not consider her early symptoms to be a serious problem or connect it to leprosy:

> After having my youngest daughter, I swelled up suddenly. I didn't know what it was. It was already because of this problem [leprosy] but I didn't know it. . . . Later it disappeared on its own—the swelling. . . . Then [I had] a burn on my leg—I burned myself [due to insensitivity]. But I didn't connect it. I thought it was normal. My husband said it wasn't normal, that I should find a doctor. . . . Now, it's not normal, I know. I didn't make the connection [Não liguei], you know?

Eugênio, seventy, said that he had spots for twenty years before a dermatologist friend suggested to him that it could be hanseníase:

> My wife would say, especially in the summer, when it was hotter . . . she would say, "You're all spotted"—spotted on my shoulders, and even my belly had spots. I thought it was from the liver. It's hard to go to the doctor, you know? I thought it was liver spots.

Liver spots (which are, incidentally, not related to actual liver function) are caused by extensive sun exposure and tend to show up more frequently with age. Gerson, twenty-three, also thought that his spots were liver spots or "because of the beach." Leprosy has very mild symptoms in its earliest stages (some paucibacillary patients never develop severe symptoms), and few patients will seek treatment if they are experiencing no pain. Because there are a host of other skin conditions in Rio de Janeiro that are worse than the spots associated with early-stage leprosy, it is understandable that people disregard the appearance of small, depigmented, painless spots on their skin. Even in cases such as Denise's, in which a patient is injured or burned because of insensitivity, if the patient feels no pain, he or she is less inclined to seek treatment.

Funguses and other minor skin problems are very prevalent among those who live in favelas, primarily in areas where there are open sewers and a lack of basic sanitation. Many people in the shantytowns are accustomed to walking barefoot or with only flip-flops. In addition, swimming in the ocean in Rio can bring all sorts of skin problems. There are several sewer lines through which treated sewage is carried out into the ocean. It is common to see beaches in Rio listed in the newspaper as unsuitable for swimming; those listed as acceptable are adjacent to the unsuitable ones. Yet during the summer, the waters of both suitable and unsuitable beaches are full of bathers and surfers. In April of 1999, a severe leak in one of the sewage pipes in Ipanema resulted in closure of the beaches. Media reports and government signs warned that swimming could result in funguses, rashes, and possibly hepatitis. Early symptoms of leprosy often resemble skin problems acquired at the beach, but because skin discolorations and changes are so common, most people delay quite a bit before going in to see a doctor.

Seeking Treatment

For people in Rio de Janeiro with health problems, there are many treatment choices. Many people attempt some form of home remedy or alternative cure before going to a hospital or health post. Others use alternative treatments in conjunction with biomedical treatment or because of frustration with biomedical care. They claim that AIDS, TB, cancer, and other diseases with prolonged treatment programs can be cured through participation in evangelical churches. A janitor I met in the favela school where I worked was a member of the Assembly of God Church, and he told me that he had seen someone cured of leprosy in his church. Based on conversations with healthcare workers and others who work with patients, it seems that the belief that leprosy can be cured in the church is common among evangelicals, although (as will be discussed below) many of the patients I interviewed did not believe that the cure could be found in religion alone.

Catholicism and Afro-Brazilian religions also offer spiritual cures for serious illnesses. In Catholicism, people with physical ailments can make *promessas* (literally, promises) to a saint to "perform some sacrificial act" in exchange for healing of their illness (Page 1995, 326). Miracle cures, brought about through a particular saint or sacred site, were also frequently reported in the news when I was in Brazil. In a Candomblé and Umbanda store in Rio de Janeiro, I asked the clerks what they would suggest for someone with lepra or other skin afflictions. They said to light a candle for Saint Lazarus or Saint Roch. In general, offerings to Omolu, the corresponding orixá to these saints, serve to prevent illness, but he is sometimes sought to heal as well. Omolu is an appealing figure in part because he represents the "wounded doctor" (Caprara 1998, 123). He is the ideal physician, who can empathize with patients because he has experienced severe illness and deformity himself. However, a curing ceremony can be quite complicated and sometimes costly, and it often involves the initiation of the sick person as *filha/filho do santo* (daughter/son of a saint).

Of the patients I interviewed, only two (of the forty-one in treatment) considered a completely religion-based cure. Jacira, forty-five, whose son was an evangelical Protestant and whose daughter was a follower of Umbanda or Candomblé (Jacira did not specify), eventually was convinced by her daughter to seek treatment and see a religious specialist:

C.W.: What did [the religious specialist] say?

JACIRA: Well, I went to her house. Then she threw some things [*búzios*—cowrie shells used for divination] for me. I respect this, but I don't like to participate. I'm afraid of getting involved in these things.

C.W.: Was it Candomblé or—?

JACIRA: I think it was . . . I had been out of work for six months and I didn't have money for hardly anything. God helped me. I didn't have any money after six months without work. [My ex-husband] pays when he wants and sometimes forgets, right? But I thought, o.k., let's go. So she said a lot of things to me. In the end, she gave me an enormous list of things I would have to buy. She said that [someone] had [cursed me] for me to die. I was afraid. . . . She gave

me this enormous list. At the time . . . I didn't even have milk to
be able to eat right.

C.W.: What things were on the list?

JACIRA: I don't know. Those things that they use, right? . . . She said,
"When you've bought all these things, I'm going to take you to the
barracão [large house, often used to refer to the *terreiro*, a center for
Umbanda or Candomblé]. You'll stay there lying down for three days.
Three days lying down? I thought, "My God, my God, how, not even
knowing this girl, how am I going to stay lying down for three days,
away from my house? Sleep three days in a place I don't even know?"
Without any understanding of the religion, you're not going to do
something you don't understand. . . . God forgive me. I liked the girl.
She said some things very fast, but I wasn't going to do them. I'm
going to have to get better with the love of God . . . I am getting better,
thank God. They [the doctors] already consider me cured.

Not being a member of the religion herself, the treatment offered
by this specialist only produced anxiety for Jacira. She was asked to
buy items she could not afford and participate in a ritual she did not
understand. However, I present her story to illustrate that members
of Afro-Brazilian religions might offer suggestions about etiology and
treatment for leprosy.

Twenty patients I interviewed (exactly half of forty patients whose
religion I recorded) were members of a denomination of an evangelical
Protestant church. In some cases, patients were encouraged to abandon
the biomedical realm altogether and focus on a spiritual solution for
a cure, as is illustrated in Sônia's narrative in chapter 6. Though the
stated position of some of these churches is sometimes to abandon
treatment when it does not seem to be effective, individual religious
leaders often take a more open-minded view, suggesting that religious
healing be supplemented with medical healing. Denise, twenty-seven,
a member of the Igreja Universal, told me:

I talked to the pastors. They said that God also cures this [han-
seníase]. He said that there is the side of the doctors and the side
of God, that I should come to church also because God cures you,

God frees you. There's medicine, things of doctors. But for God, nothing's impossible. Because God is the doctor of doctors.

Many patients also negotiated their own interpretation of what it meant to be cured by Jesus by seeing doctors as emissaries of Jesus. Lorenzo, forty-two, who had not yet received a diagnosis of leprosy but had completed the diagnostic tests, admitted he was worried, but if he did have leprosy, he knew it was curable: "I'll do my part. I'm going to the doctor. The doctor does his part. What the doctor can't do, then it's [up to] Jesus." Though a strong believer in the power of his evangelical church, he also believed in the medical treatment available. Among patients, understandings of the curability of leprosy had less to do with popular or folk models of leprosy and more to do with how the disease is presented to patients in the medical encounter, which is the topic of the next chapter.

There are also many home remedies available for lepra, although none have been proven scientifically to kill the leprosy bacilli. Many of these remedies are related to Afro-Brazilian religious practice, but people of many different religions in Brazil employ these types of treatments outside of a ritual context. All over the city of Rio de Janeiro, one can find vendors selling herbs and plants of different kinds that can be used for various ailments. On the sidewalk in front of the Santa Casa de Misericórdia hospital in Rio, for example, there is often a vendor selling medicinal plants laid out on a large sheet, offering patients a potential alternative or supplement to hospital treatment. During *feiras livres* (open-air markets) held in various *praças* (plazas) throughout Rio on different days of the week, abundant fresh fruit, fish, and spices are sold, and a few vendors have tables piled high with a variety of leaves and bark. Plant parts are also sold in packages at many stands and newspaper kiosks. I approached several of these vendors in order to find out what treatment alternatives are available for patients, specifically the popular names of the plants that are sold for skin problems or lepra. When I first talked to a vendor at a feira livre in Ipanema and asked if he had treatments for skin diseases or skin blemishes (*doenças de pele ou manchas na pele*), he pulled out a few bunches of cut plants from under the pile. I followed up by mentioning the terms *lepra* and *hanseníase* specifically and was given more leaves and bark. Vendors in other parts of the city gave me several other plants and told me the popular names (including *urucum, erva de bicho, erva de São João, erva de Santa Maria, espinheira santa, amor do campo,* and *aroeira*). Notably, urucum, or annatto (*Bixa orellana*) was studied by Brazilian scientists in the early twentieth century as a possible leprosy treatment (Souza-Araújo 1948, plate 38). A leprosy patient interviewed by Claro (1995, 75) in Rio de Janeiro said that she used *aroeira* (generally the popular name for *Schinus terebinthefolius*) to make a bath. The patient told her, "There's no better remedy for these inflammations than aroeira. My legs were one wound that just opened up. I got better with this herb. It was the medications and the aroeira."

Several magazines, booklets, and journals of home remedies and herbal cures are sold in newspaper kiosks in Rio de Janeiro. I did not encounter one that mentioned a specific nonmedical cure for lepra or hanseníase. However, some offer cures for symptoms of leprosy and other skin ailments. For example, in the booklet *Remédios Caseiros* (Home Remedies), the following recommendations are given for general spots (*manchas na pele*) and for *pano*, a popular name for vitiligo:

> Apply daily sugar mixed with lemon juice. Wash the area with tea from leaves of *celidônia* [probably *Chelidonium majus*]. Pulverize basil until all the juice is extracted. Mix the juice with alcohol. Soak a cotton ball in the mixture and rub it over the spots. They will soon disappear. (Quintão 1998, 7)

Patients have fairly easy access to these popular magazines, which are relatively inexpensive, and some patients might try some of these remedies before visiting a health post.

Psychic surgery, or "spiritual" surgery, is another option available to some in Brazil. Sidney Greenfield (1999) describes spiritual surgery as performed by a specialist who believed he was the reincarnation of the spirit of a famous surgeon. A psychologist and volunteer at MORHAN told me that this option was available for patients in Rio de Janeiro, although she did not know of any cases in which leprosy patients sought help from spiritual surgeons. A specialist she was aware of in Rio also performed surgery as the reincarnation of a particular spirit. She told me that the specialist believes that "it's only the spirit that can eliminate illness," working through the physical incarnation of the specialist.

All of the above alternative treatments demonstrate the plurality of medicines and healing techniques that are available to people with leprosy in Brazil. Although from a biomedical point of view none of these techniques is an effective treatment for curing leprosy, it is possible that some forms of treatment, particularly the plant-based treatments, are useful for leprosy reaction and for other complications associated with leprosy. Treatments of a supernatural nature may also have a powerful effect on the immune system and on the overall health of the person. On the other hand, some alternative treatments can interfere with and cause complications with multidrug therapy.

In seeking a cure for leprosy, most patients I spoke with were adamant about sticking to the prescribed treatment plan at the clinic. Alternative medicines included creams and lotions bought in a pharmacy (but not prescribed by the doctor) and teas and baths made from medicinal herbs. The small percentage of patients who said they tried alternative treatments may not reflect the true picture of patient self-medication or self-treatment for leprosy in Rio. Although Claro (1995) suggested that the use of herbal medicines is diminishing in the large cities of Brazil, in favor of pharmaceutical medicines, I think more patients use alternative treatments than are reflected in my sample. Most patients I interviewed were being seen at a treatment facility where patients generally claimed to have a great deal of faith in the physicians and the treatment. The interviews were conducted there as well, so patients may not have wanted to admit to physicians that they had tried alternative treatments. Another problem was that the terminology I used, "*tratamentos alternativos*," was not well understood by patients. Only late in my interviewing process did I realize that "*remédios caseiros*" (home remedies) was more clearly interpreted by patients.

Pamela, forty-eight, said that she tried several home remedies before and during the initial stages of her treatment. She tried teas, baths, and various lotions; one bath she prepared, using medicinal plants, "burned a lot." One patient I spoke with informally brought in a small box to show to the doctor at a leprosy referral center. The label on the side said "*banha peixe elêtrico*," supposedly an extract of the electric eel. He brought out small white papers from the box and rubbed one on his skin to demonstrate. The pamphlet that came with the box said that it can be used for neuritis, among other things; he was using it for the nerve pain in his hands, perhaps as a stimulant for circulation. In 2005, I found another brand of electric eel extract in the form of a waxy balm, in a medicinal products stand at the Feira de São Cristovão, a weekly fair in Rio that celebrates the culture of the Northeast region of Brazil.

The healthcare workers and volunteers I interviewed told me that patients often use home remedies, which mostly consist of natural medicines such as herbs and other plants, from which teas for drinking or baths are made. A MORHAN volunteer told me that floral therapy (*terapia floral*), based on the use of flower-based substances, "which is in fashion right now," was sometimes reported in patient self-help groups. Future research might be useful to determine which alternative treatments could help patients and which might complicate treatment or react negatively with multidrug therapy and other medications.

The Flexibility of Patient Explanatory Models of Leprosy

A theme that emerged from the narratives I collected was that the explanatory models that patients held were far from fixed. In contrast to an idea of statically or firmly held beliefs that interfered with a person's willingness to take steps toward getting well, the leprosy-affected individuals I met and spoke with were very flexible in terms of their views about their illness (White 2005). They were willing to accept what their physicians told them about it being a curable disease and its person-to-person mode of transmission, for example. At the same time, awareness of the biomedical model did not mean that patients entirely abandoned previously held beliefs about the body and health in general or about leprosy or infectious disease specifically. Like anyone who has experienced a complicated or chronic illness, the people I met had, for the most part, thought quite a bit about different aspects of their disease and often come up with their own unique models for understanding it, which were constantly in flux. What I found was that patients' explanatory models about their illness evolved and changed during different phases of their disease and as a result of their contact with healthcare professionals, family members, friends, employers, and others. Folk and scientific models were not mutually exclusive for patients. A person might simultaneously believe that God is responsible for curing them and that God works through the doctors and the medications that have been made available to them.

Why care about folk models or explanatory models of disease? Some would argue that any beliefs that patients have that are "wrong" or do not match with the biomedical view are irrelevant or relevant only in terms of potentially interfering with treatment. However, there are many reasons why it is important for public health officials, policy makers, and healthcare workers to understand both folk and explanatory models of leprosy. Folk models may impact patient treatment-seeking behavior to some extent; patients may wait to seek care because early leprosy symptoms do not match the folk model of leprosy in their severity. Folk models may affect how stigma is constructed and acted upon by patients, their families, other members of their communities, and their employers. These beliefs can also influence patient mental and emotional health and well-being. However, because individual patients' explanatory models are subject to their personal experience with leprosy, physicians and other healthcare workers can influence these models. Every aspect of what I call the "medical encounter," the subject of the next chapter, is important in shaping and altering patient explanatory models that can either improve patients' overall experience with leprosy or exacerbate problems created by this disease.

4

The Medical Encounter

Seeking a Cure, Seeking Wellness

In many ways, Brazil is ahead of much of the rest of the world in its approach to health care. Since 1996, for example, Brazil has been a world leader in putting pressure on pharmaceutical companies to lower their prices for drugs for HIV/AIDS treatment by producing their own generic versions of these drugs. Healthcare services are, by order of law, provided to all Brazilians free of charge. This has been true in Brazil since the inauguration of the Sistema Único de Saúde (SUS, Single or Universal Health System) in 1988. The law that established the SUS states that it was created "with the aim of changing the situation of inequality of access to health care, making it obligatory to provide public health services to every citizen and prohibiting charging for services under any pretext" (my translation, from Sistema Única de Saúde 2004). However, Brazil's economic commitment to public health is less impressive, with a low percentage of the gross domestic product spent on health care relative to other industrialized nations and to other nations in a similar stage of development. Most middle-class and upper-class individuals do not use these services and instead usually purchase health insurance and go to private clinics and hospital (Alves and Timmins 2003).

Inadequate spending on public health contributes to periodic shortages of medications, of proper equipment, and of physicians and healthcare staff who are interested in working permanently or full time in the public health system. Extended waiting times for treatment at public health posts are also common (Alves and Timmins 2003). Newspaper and television reports in Rio frequently contain stories of malpractice and poor treatment that patients and their families receive at public health hospitals. At the end of March 1999, for example, there was a shortage of doctors throughout Rio de Janeiro's public health facilities. A physicians' union that was responsible for paying its doctors had not paid them for three months, so many of the doctors went on strike. The result was hugely understaffed hospitals and negligence of even emergency cases. A nurse interviewed for the story, reported in the *Jornal do Brasil* newspaper, confirmed that some patients had not eaten for days because there had been no doctors available to prescribe special diets for them (Bittencourt 1999, 17). Another publicized example of the problems related to the strike was the case of Pedro Ricardo Mendes, who died of a cerebral hemorrhage in the Hospital Getúlio Vargas, in Rio de Janeiro, thirty-four hours after arriving at the emergency room. At this hospital, they were not able to find him a spot in the intensive care ward, so his sister-in-law drove all over town trying to find a place for him. Upon returning to the hospital, she could not find the patient and was obliged to have his physician awakened in order to get approval for transfer to another hospital. The physician, reportedly angry at being disturbed and complaining he had not been paid for months, refused to approve the patient's transfer. She sought the help of another physician, who claimed it was out of his hands. The sister-in-law said she lost her temper and threatened to call the press, and it was only then that the patient was placed on a respirator, though without proper early care, he died (17). Several anthropologists (Goldstein 2003; Gregg 2003; Scheper-Hughes 1992) who have done fieldwork in Brazilian favelas, where residents rely primarily on public services for health care, have described abuses or inadequate care experienced by patients and their families at public health posts.

These incidents cannot be understood simply as the result of a lack of empathy on the part of doctors. There is little incentive in Brazil for physicians to work in public health when private practice is so much more lucrative and less stressful. Many of the better physicians, save those who are genuinely dedicated to public service, do not devote their careers to working in public health clinics. Conditions are poor and resources are limited at public health posts, and doctors and nurses at these facilities are typically overworked. Thus, many public health clinics are staffed largely by medical interns, who are required to do some work within the SUS during their training. The perceptions that some middle-class and upper-class health professionals have of people from poor communities also affect the experience of patients at public health clinics. People from the favelas and other low-income neighborhoods sometimes are viewed as simple, ignorant, and unable to process information about their own health and bodies. The majority of healthcare workers I observed in leprosy referral centers treated patients with kindness and care, in contrast to patients' reported experiences at other health posts. However, even in these treatment centers, a few healthcare workers regarded patients as untrustworthy, in terms of the information they provided to physicians about themselves, and unable to handle certain types of complex medical information. In particular, some of the interns who passed through the clinic exhibited a somewhat disparaging attitude toward patients. On one occasion, I discussed with an intern my research finding that many patients who have been through MDT counseled other patients about the experience while waiting for their appointment outside of the clinic. He was quite skeptical of the value of these patient conversations and scoffed, "How can a patient help another patient?" implying that only physicians had the power, authority, and knowledge to help someone who is ill. While this did not reflect the attitude of most of the physicians and nurses I met and worked with, patients often related stories to me of other health posts where they felt that they had been treated poorly.

Fieldwork in a Medical Setting

Since the bulk of my observations and interviews took place in public health settings rather than in a circumscribed community, many of my informants or "key cultural consultants" (Kottak 2004) were the regular nurses, physicians, and social workers at the health posts where I spent most of my time. I established a good rapport with many healthcare workers, and most of the people I met were very interested in my project and eager to encourage patients to talk with me. In 1998–1999, leprosy was treated at only a handful of referral centers around the city of Rio. The permanent staff at these clinics were committed and passionate about the work they were doing and were well liked by most of the patients with whom I talked. In many ways, these leprosy treatment facilities did not necessarily provide a representative picture of the experience of the public healthcare system in Brazil. The referral center where I conducted most of my interviews received substantial funding from national and international sources, so salaries were higher than at most health posts. Both my observations and patient narratives confirmed that patients were treated kindly, and as "human beings," as patients noted. The high quality of interactions between healthcare workers and patients at these clinics helped to create a level of trust that carried over into my relationships with the patients I met.

I spent time observing and talking to patients and staff at four different treatment centers for leprosy in Rio de Janeiro and its suburbs, but the majority of my time was spent at one outpatient treatment facility, where medical research was also conducted. One of the patients I interviewed, Humberto, fifty, praised the staff there and contrasted them to the staff at many health posts:

HUMBERTO: I was never received in any other place with the care that these people have for us. It's marvelous care. They are honest people. Really humane. I've never been to another hospital like it, where I was well treated as I have been here and continue to be today. Every time I come here, the people are the same, the same style, the same manner of speaking with us. I think it's marvelous. We need more of that in our country.

C.W.: What do you think of the health posts? Are they that way also?

HUMBERTO: The health posts are very different. . . . Outside it's very different because they don't insist on taking care of the sick. They come in, ask what I have, hand me medicines, send me away or give me an injection. They don't try to reach me to know if there's a need for better understanding. It's very difficult. We don't see this around here. So after I came here, I never wanted to go to another place. I won't go to another hospital—for anything. Only if they direct me to another place, I'll go.

The atmosphere among the permanent staff was extremely conge-
nial, and I felt very welcomed there as a researcher. One nurse always
greeted me with a giant smile and addressed me in dramatic fashion
as "Cassandra Rios" after a twentieth-century Brazilian author of erotic
novels. At first I was unsure what to think about this, but I soon realized it was intended with affection. I was invited to show up any time
when they had clinic hours, and I was allowed to come and go at my
convenience. I would sometimes accompany the clinic staff to lunch at
a nearby *comida ao kilo* (buffet-style, in which the price is determined
by the weight of your food) cafeteria. I would share espressolike coffees
(*cafezinhos*) with the staff at the clinic, and once in a while, I would
hitch a ride home with one of the physicians.

Shortly after the permanent staff got to know me, they started to
alert me to patients they thought I should meet. Typically when I was
conducting interviews and observations at the clinic, I was unable
to meet every patient who came for their appointment, but I could
count on nurses, doctors, and social workers to introduce me to individuals whose cases were particularly interesting or whose experiences
with leprosy had been complicated. I was always invited to enter the
exam areas and social workers' offices, although there were several
times when I felt my presence was somewhat invasive for the patient.
Although I made it clear to the clinic staff and to patients that I was
not a doctor, they often were interested in discussing patients' cases
with me in complex medical terms, as if I were one of the many interns
that came through the clinic. In this way, I did become proficient at
distinguishing the diagnostic symptoms of leprosy from those of other
diseases. I often felt uncomfortable if, as was often the case, a physician
would insist that I remain in an exam room as the patient removed all
or part of their clothing. I was often concerned that my presence in the
exam room made me a party to the further objectification of the patient
as a "diseased body." However, I felt that by refusing to participate in
this aspect of the clinical experience, I risked offending the healthcare
workers who so generously included me in clinic life.

Because a steady stream of medical students came to the clinic
for short internships, I had to explain my presence in the clinic with
relative frequency. Occasionally, an intern would ask me for advice

about a patient's treatment plan (which, of course, I could not give). Patients would describe symptoms or complications to me that they had not shared with the doctor but that seemed to be significant, and I would sometimes act as a liaison between the two. I talked to patients during biopsies and painful skin scrapings, sometimes holding a patient's hand and discussing his or her pain or difficulty with the experience.

I came up with several strategies that allowed me to participate (as an observer) in medical exams but at the same time separate myself, in the minds of both patients and healthcare workers, as "not a doctor," despite often being introduced as *Doutora* (Doctor) Cassandra. I remembered that Maxine Margolis, a Brazilianist and anthropologist who headed my master's thesis committee, told me how she was surprised to be consistently addressed as "doutora" well before she had received a PhD. In Brazil, a bachelor's degree is sufficient to gain this title. Although I may have been a doutora in Brazil, I emphasized that I was not a *médica* (medical doctor). I made a point not to wear the white typically worn by healthcare workers throughout Brazil. Doctors, interns, and nurses at the clinics I visited wore different varieties of white pants and white shirts, along with a white lab coat while on duty. Since patients were generally positioned opposite the physicians at a small desk, I would sit on a stool to the side of the desk, in a seemingly more neutral space.

In order to open up a dialogue with a patient, I would wait while the doctor was either busily writing or in another room, and I would ask the patient where he or she lived. Then I would introduce myself and say, "I'm not a doctor. I'm an anthropologist from the United States doing research on hanseníase and the problems that patients have with hanseníase." I would briefly explain that I was interested in cultural aspects of Hansen's disease, though I was never sure that the people I interviewed fully understood what the role of an anthropologist was. However, the job of "anthropologist" in contemporary Brazil is more a part of the public discourse than it is in the United States. There are several anthropologists, such as Roberto DaMatta and Darcy Ribeiro, who have often been featured in the media for their work with indigenous populations in Brazil and on Brazilian popular culture. Ribeiro was also a prominent politician in Brazil in the years leading up to his death in 1997.

I believe that establishing my status as an outsider, in terms of being an American anthropologist rather than a Brazilian physician, allowed patients to feel more comfortable speaking with me. They also may have felt there were certain things I would not understand as a non-Brazilian and they needed to explain to me. Even in informal conversations, patients often opened up to me about not only health-related issues but also their daily lives at work and home. Thus, through both my formal and informal interviews and through my observations of interactions between healthcare workers and patients, I learned about some aspects of the medical encounter that were problematic for patients in their quest for a diagnosis, for treatment, and for a cure for their illness.

Communicating across Class Lines

One of the primary concerns within medical anthropology that has emerged in the last few decades is the quality of the interaction between healthcare workers and patients. This relationship, particularly between physicians and patients, is typically an unbalanced one, as healthcare workers are the holders of an exclusive or "authoritative" knowledge about the body and about health and illness that is learned in the setting of medical school or other forms of specialized medical training (Good and Good 1993). Challenging or questioning this knowledge can be difficult for even a college-educated individual who is not trained in a biomedical field. In settings such as public health posts or hospitals in Rio de Janeiro, the gap in shared experience and knowledge between healthcare workers and patients is made more extreme by the sharp class and cultural differences that usually exist between these groups. Although I met nurses and medical assistants and technicians who could be classified as solidly middle class or lower-middle class, most, if not all, of the physicians and medical interns I met came from the middle, upper-middle, or upper classes. Class differences translate to drastically different life experiences, and some healthcare workers do not have firsthand knowledge of the challenges of everyday life faced by many of the patients they treat. Norms of social interaction between the elite and the lower class, between boss and worker, or between the household head and the domestic worker are mirrored in relationships between doctors and patients. These class divisions are unconsciously maintained by both physicians and patients. Patients defer to doctors and refer to them as "o doutor" or *o senhor/a senhora* (sir/madam) whereas physicians frequently call patients by their first name. I noticed that some physicians, who also seemed to have an excellent rapport with patients, attempted to break these boundaries by using the respectful terms of "o senhor" and "a senhora" with patients.

Boundaries that structure the rules of communication across classes often resulted in patients being hesitant to ask questions or volunteer information about their condition. During interviews and informal conversations, patients would tell me about a physical problem they had, and when I asked if they had told the doctor about it, they said no. On one occasion, I was waiting in an exam room with a twelve-year-old girl (the patient) and her grandmother, when the grandmother told me that the girl had rheumatic fever three years ago and was still taking medications for it. She had not told the physician about this, so we both told him when he returned, and it seemed to make a difference in his plan of action for her. If physicians are aware that patients (or caregivers) may not have the same perception about what information is important to the patient's case, or if they are aware that patients will not readily volunteer information, they might consider asking more specific questions before beginning treatment. Some physicians I spoke with felt that it was the patient's responsibility to make his or her problems known. Yet when patients did speak up to ask questions or discuss their own health, they sometimes met with frustration. For example, Renata, thirty-six, told me that she did not know the names of some of her medications because, she said, "I don't like to ask, you know? I don't like to ask questions. Because sometimes people say, 'Oh, you're a pain.'" Her experience of going against the norms of social interaction by attempting to gain access to some of the knowledge held by health-care workers was perceived (or at least she felt that it was perceived) as causing trouble. Renata was particularly frustrated with interns who she felt did not listen to her or trust her to know how the medications were working for her. She liked the permanent doctors who had been there for some time, but, she said:

> It's just that with these inexperienced doctors who come here, I think it's totally different. They are just learning. . . . So the other day I said to [one of the permanent doctors], "One says one thing, the other says another, who am I going to follow in the end?"

Renata had an argument with one of the interns about how many sedatives she was taking. She told me she was aware of how medications were going to affect her:

> I know my body, understand? I know if something is not going to cause me problems. If I take three sedatives, I know it's not going to hurt me—She [the intern] said I can't, but I take them because my psychiatrist prescribed them for me. . . . Should I stay up stressed all night?

When patients are given information that contradicts their own experience with medications or with treatment, without further explanation, they feel frustrated. Particularly after going through years of treatment, patients become more aware of their bodies, as Renata said, and know what to expect from certain medications.

I tried to note not just the verbal communication that took place, but also the physical interactions that were necessary in treating patients. Physical interactions began with diagnosis, when patients were often asked to remove their clothes so that the physician could view any lesions or skin patches. Undressing made some patients feel awkward, and the situation was complicated further when the physician or other people in the exam room were of the opposite sex. I observed physicians telling relatives to leave the room, particularly if the relative was not a husband or wife of the patient. However, nurses and interns sometimes walked in and out while patients were undressed. This aspect of examination and diagnosis is common in biomedical settings worldwide, particularly in teaching hospitals and clinics. Xavier, thirty-two, complained about this aspect of diagnosis. He was examined at a hospital before being referred to the health post where I interviewed him, and he told me, "I know that I was in the exam room without clothes for more than an hour. Air-conditioning. Terrible cold. Every-one wanted to look at me. All of the doctors wanted to look at me." The clinic where I spent most of my times also had air-conditioning units, and I noticed that several patients, particularly those who came in with fevers to begin with, shivered throughout the exam as they sat partially or fully unclothed.

I frequently observed physicians examining a patient for the edifi-cation of a group of interns, discussing the patient's case and pointing out his or her lesions. Sometimes parts of patients' bodies were pho-tographed for educational slide presentations or journal articles. After nearly a year of observing such interactions, perhaps I became inured to the lack of privacy that patients were afforded in public health clin-ics. I became aware of this when, in 2005, I brought students who were part of my study-abroad program to a health post where leprosy was treated. The physicians at the clinic asked a patient, a man in his thir-ties or forties, to sit in front of the group of nearly twenty-five students while an intern conducted sensitivity tests on his hands and feet. The presentation of the man's symptoms was quite clinical, and though the intern asked him politely before each relatively painless procedure, the man appeared uncomfortable. Some of my students were quite shocked, saying that the incident brought them to tears, whereas I had become accustomed to witnessing this type of exam. In a class session the following day, students debated the pedagogical pros and cons of such a learning experience and wondered if the man had been coerced. I assured them that his permission was requested, as I had personally told the man just before he entered the room that it was full of *gringos* and he did not have to come in if he did not want to, after which he laughed and consented to the presentation. But as a few students wisely pointed out, he may still have felt coerced, considering that those who asked him to participate were in a position of authority and in charge of his care. My students, coming primarily from middle- or upper-class backgrounds in the United States and elsewhere, were used to what they saw as their rights as patients being carefully observed, although some could recall episodes of illness in their lives where specialists or interns had been brought in to comment on their case. As biomedicine is currently structured, it may seem difficult to balance the needs and rights of patients with the demands of teaching and learning diagnostic signs and treatment strategies. This rehumanization of the patient is one of the challenges that medical professionals face around the world and is an important factor in the establishment of trust between physicians and patients.

Misdiagnosis and Late Detection

As I discussed in the first chapter, I once thought that patient abandonment of treatment would be the top problem in leprosy control. The more I talked to patients, NGO representatives, and healthcare workers about these issues, the more I began to think that delays in disease detection, either through patients' delays in seeking treatment or through repeated misdiagnosis by physicians, was a more significant problem. Late detection contributes to the spread of leprosy, as an undiagnosed individual with multibacillary leprosy exhales a number of leprosy bacilli with every breath. In addition, the longer a person goes without treatment, the more likely he or she is to have complications related to the disease. Early detection has been suggested to be more important than regular treatment in the prevention of disabilities (Rao et al. 1996). In other words, a patient who has had symptoms of leprosy for several years without receiving treatment will be more likely to develop a disability whether or not he or she adheres faithfully to treatment.

In addition to the continued transmission of the disease and to an increased likelihood of disabilities in patients, late detection due to misdiagnosis creates much anxiety for patients. Leprosy is generally underdiagnosed in Brazil. In South Asia, some have suggested that the opposite form of misdiagnosis seems to be equally problematic. Keith Skillicorn (1998), who has worked as a missionary with leprosy patients in Bangladesh and India, observed that a diagnosis of leprosy when the patient actually has another disease or problem is common and quite harmful to the patient's well-being in the community because the stigma associated with leprosy is very strong. Doctors there are more liable to jump to the conclusion that patients with a variety of skin conditions have leprosy, so Skillicorn has cautioned against overdiagnosis. By contrast, in Brazil, doctors commonly misdiagnose people with leprosy as having a number of other conditions. One problem with diagnosis is that leprosy can take many forms, and the lesions that occur in different forms of the disease can be confused with symptoms of many other illnesses. A second problem is that the folk model of the symptoms of leprosy (rotting flesh, severe deformity, loss of limbs) is often the only model doctors are familiar with if they have not been trained in leprosy diagnosis. Thus, many doctors do not identify leprosy until the disease has developed to the point where patients will be permanently disabled. A Brazilian epidemiologist and physician I interviewed for my research told me that many doctors "think that a patient has leprosy only when he's completely deformed. They do not understand that leprosy is not like the preconceived notions of it. It presents itself in many forms." Also, leprosy is often mistakenly considered by physicians to be a dermatological condition, he said, when it is really an infectious disease that affects the nerves and also manifests itself in lesions on the skin, but it is not technically a "skin disease." Physicians, he told me, need to be better trained to spot problems in nerve function and sensitivity that may be related to leprosy. Another point he brought up was that physicians receive very little training on the diseases that are most common in Brazil among the poor, stating that "it's inexcusable that our Brazilian doctors don't know leprosy, tuberculosis, malnutrition, diarrhea." It is true that leprosy can resemble other illnesses. However, it was apparent from my own observations that minimal training is required to distinguish most forms of leprosy from other diseases; although I have no clinical medical training, I felt confident within the first few weeks of my fieldwork that I could identify some of the most common signs of leprosy. Insensitivity in a light-colored or reddish patch of skin usually distinguishes leprosy from other skin problems. Boy and Girl Scouts in several countries where leprosy is endemic have been trained in identifying suspected cases of the disease (World Organization of the Scouting Movement 2005). Brazilian medical students could easily be trained to recognize the most common diagnostic signs of the disease. A health official I interviewed told me that the Municipal Secretary (Office) of Health of Rio de Janeiro has offered several training positions in leprosy diagnosis and treatment in Rio de Janeiro, but these positions usually went unfilled. She said that

this was partly because the number of hours interns are given for training is low and partly because the Secretary of Health is more interested
in the number of patients that doctors or interns see than the quality
of their service or of their training. In addition, she said, many interns
were not interested in learning more about a disease that is prevalent
among the poor and generally treated in public healthcare clinics,
where physicians are very poorly remunerated. She said that doctors in
public health were earning around R$460 per month at a health post,
although some may have positions at more than one health post. At
the time of my interview with the health official, R$460 was around
U.S.$250 a month.

The Municipal Secretary (Office) of Health of Rio de Janeiro com-
piled a list of some of the situations in which the medical community
loses the opportunity for a diagnosis. For example, patients may go to
a clinic where their symptoms are not recognized or where healthcare
workers do not schedule them for a return visit; the health post staff
may not recognize leprosy, or they may not have the diagnostic tools
to test for it; patients are misdiagnosed and treated for another illness;
patients may not have access to or know where they can find treatment;
and patients may go in for treatment of another problem but have
symptoms of leprosy (that the patient has not been concerned with),
and the medical staff does not recognize these symptoms (Secretária
Municipal de Saúde do Rio de Janeiro 1997).

The patients I interviewed told me about their often long and
circuitous path to finding a diagnosis of their condition. Eighteen of
them (about 40 percent of the patients I interviewed) had received a
misdiagnosis of their condition. Other studies of leprosy patients in
Brazil also reveal fairly high percentages of patients who have been
misdiagnosed. Queiroz and Puntel (1997) note that close to 90 percent
of the thirty-three patients they interviewed in Campinas, São Paulo,
had been misdiagnosed at least once before finding out what they had.
In Claro's (1995) study of forty-five leprosy patients in Rio de Janeiro,
twelve (29 percent) had experienced misdiagnosis of their disease, and
two others (5 percent) were told they had nothing wrong with them.

Among patients I met and interviewed, physicians had misdiagnosed their illness as one or more of several different conditions,

including fungus, allergy or rash, arthritis and other joint inflammation problems, diabetes, syphilis, and circulation or heart problems. One of the more common misdiagnoses was of *micose* (fungus), for which patients were often prescribed an antibiotic or antifungal cream, which usually had no effect. In some cases, the cream would be effective temporarily, but then lesions or spots would reappear shortly thereafter. Walter, twenty-eight, had his first symptoms of leprosy when he was eighteen but said he did not connect the symptoms to a problem at first. When he did seek treatment, he went to a health post and could not get a diagnosis. Then he went to a private doctor, who said he had a fungus. Flávia, forty-seven, said she went to many dermatologists in the suburb of Nova Iguaçu, where she lived, but that she did not get the correct diagnosis. For two years, she was treated with several different skin creams that did not help the spot she had on her leg. Eventually, she read more about leprosy at the library in the high school where she worked and thus managed to diagnose herself. The diagnosis of a leprosy skin patch as a fungus most likely represents a failure on the physician's part to test the lesion for sensitivity.

Doctors also frequently confuse leprosy symptoms with allergic reaction. Wilson, thirty-six, received this type of misdiagnosis:

> I went to the community doctor. I had those red spots. He gave me medicines for—he thought it was an allergy. . . . He gave me antibiotics, and it [spots] disappeared within the hour. I thought it was taken care of. But three days later, it returned. I went to another doctor. He prescribed to me a medicine from the same laboratory but with a different name, a little different, also for allergy. I took it, I was fine. Three days went by, and everything came back.

Because *M. leprae* is a bacillus, general antibiotics may have a temporary effect on clearing up symptoms, but once the antibiotics are out of the patient's system, the symptoms return in full force. Beth, nineteen, was also told she had an allergy:

> The first time I went to the doctor, there on the Ilha [do Governador], at the Fundão, where they have that hospital there, they

said that it was an allergy, and they put a cream on it. And it
didn't help anything. Again, they gave me a cream. I put more
and more on and nothing happened. . . . Later I went to find out
exactly what this was because I talked with the doctor, and he said
I didn't have anything. Always the same thing [in terms of not getting a diagnosis]. And [symptoms] were appearing even more.

Many patients sought the help of physicians repeatedly over a long
period of time before getting a diagnosis. Humberto, fifty, had symptoms (primarily lesions) for about fifteen years before diagnosis. He
had been to various health posts, "but they never detected anything
interesting. When they examined me, they would just give me some
medicine that didn't resolve the problem at all." Again, because the
symptoms were mild, doctors did not associate his problem with leprosy. Fernando, twenty at the time of my interview, was misdiagnosed
twice and categorically told he did not have leprosy. He was a state
karate champion and at first thought that problems with his knee,
including pain, a tingling sensation, and numbness, might be due to
the physical stress of training and breaking boards.

I went to the health post in 1996 to see what it was, in Nova
Iguaçu. There, the staff told me it was not hanseníase. Then [a
month later] I went to the health post in Belford Roxo. The doctor
examined the spots here and she said that it wasn't hanseníase,
it was dermatitis. She looked at my knee [where he was having a
lot of pain] and said it was not hanseníase.

Fernando thus went another year before his aunt brought him to the
leprosy referral center where he completed his treatment. He continued to experience numbness on the spot on his knee and eventually got
a correct diagnosis. He suffered from severe leprosy reaction toward the
end of his treatment, possibly because of the delayed diagnosis. Jacira,
forty-five, said that she first went to the doctor after having terrible
pains in her feet. She was given an injection and "many medications,
but it didn't get better." Then she saw an orthopedist, followed by a
diabetes specialist, but she continued to have problems, until she was
finally sent to a referral center for leprosy. Janete, forty-one, found out

that she was not the only one who had a difficult time getting a diagnosis by talking to other patients outside the clinic:

> A lot of people I converse with here went to several places, ran around to different places, spent years taking the wrong medicines. It hurt them a lot because when they arrive here, they're already in a well-advanced stage of the disease.

The delay in diagnosis was very frustrating for patients I talked to and contributed to anxiety, clinical depression, and feelings of despair. The two contributing factors in late detection are patient delay and physician misdiagnosis or nondiagnosis. Patient delay is somewhat harder to control, although increased education and awareness can help some patients to self-diagnose and come in for treatment earlier. Once patients with symptoms make it to a clinic or health post, physicians need to be able to diagnose leprosy so that patients can be treated as soon as possible to avoid disabilities and, in multibacillary patients, to stop transmitting the disease to others as soon as possible.

Diagnostic Procedures

Diagnostic testing for leprosy can cause much distress to patients. Some of the first-time patients I talked to informally had these tests performed on them without knowing what they were being tested for and before they received orientation about the disease. Some of the diagnostic procedures were painful. The skin smear test, or *baciloscopia,* involves the collection of tissue ("lymph," as it was explained to me, rather than blood) from areas of the body where the bacilli are likely to reside. These areas include the earlobes, elbows, knees, and lesions themselves. Though upon first glance, this procedure seems simple enough, many patients find it very painful. The patient is directed to sit with his back toward the nurse or other healthcare worker who performs the procedure. A scalpel is used to make a tiny perforation, first on one of the earlobes. Usually a bit of bleeding occurs. After the perforation is made, the nurse scrapes the area several times with the scalpel until a visible amount of material can be collected and placed on a slide. The process is repeated on the other ear lobe, both elbows, and both knees. One of the six areas would be excluded if a skin scraping could be taken from a lesion.

Because of the small amount of bleeding that sometimes occurs from this procedure, a nurse would have small strips of white medical paper tape with a bit of cotton underneath ready to fold over the earlobes and place on the elbows and knees. Thus the patient would leave the clinic with numerous small pieces of paper-tape bandages, including "*brincos*" (earrings), as the nurses and patients referred to the tape on the earlobes. The initial perforation caused most patients I observed to wince. Different patients had different reactions to the series of skin scrapings; many individuals, adults and children alike, started to cry during the procedure, partly from pain and partly, perhaps, from the stressful nature of their situation. However, the painfulness of this procedure should not be underestimated. In patients experiencing leprosy reaction at the time of testing, the skin is very sensitive and the slightest touch may be excruciatingly painful. Again, because these procedures are often performed on patients before they get their diagnosis and before they have received any medical information about leprosy, many patients do not know why the test is being performed. If they do not obtain proper assurances from clinic staff, they may leave the clinic frightened and traumatized.

Another diagnostic technique is the biopsy. At the different clinics where I conducted observations, biopsies were a standard procedure. The first leprosy-related diagnostic procedure I witnessed in 1995 during preliminary research was a punch biopsy of an elderly man with an advanced case of multibacillary leprosy. Having witnessed no medical procedures performed on anyone but myself, I stood close to the open window breathing fresh air as I tried not to faint. They gave the man an injection of anesthetic first, and then used a narrow, hollow metal tube that was pushed deep into his skin at the site of a lesion to collect a tissue sample to test for the presence of leprosy bacilli. Most biopsies I witnessed were conducted after a local anesthetic injection was given, although in some cases, the patients have no feeling in the area of the biopsy because of nerve damage from leprosy. One social worker I interviewed, however, told me that patients complained to her that doctors performed biopsies without anesthesia at a health post in another municipality. The social worker questioned the doctor in charge, who assured her that anesthesia was used. It is possible that patients confused biopsies with skin scrapings, which are certainly painful and also involve puncturing the skin, and patients are given no anesthetic for this procedure. They may also have associated the biopsy with the pain of the initial injection, but it is also possible that, in some cases, anesthetic was not used or that it was ineffective.

Besides the pain that they can cause, biopsies create significant scars, sometimes half an inch in diameter. Biopsies of the nerve that are taken from the hand or arm produce deep wounds. Humberto, fifty, said that one biopsy he had was very painful and complained, "I always leave here with more holes than a sieve." At one clinic where I engaged in observations, doctors discussed doing a biopsy of a lesion or skin patch on the face of a young girl of seven or eight years old. The social worker stepped in and protested that if it was not absolutely necessary they should not do it because she was so young and pretty and would have that scar forever; it was decided not to do the biopsy after all. The consequences of a biopsy for a person's appearance and subsequent self-image should be considered when assessing the medical need for performing the procedure.

Another social worker I interviewed talked to me of her concerns about both biopsies and skin smears. She thought that because many health posts provide training for medical students and interns, some procedures might be overused for educational purposes:

> There are patients who leave upset, afraid, when they leave the exam room where they do the biopsy or the skin smear. This is one thing you traditionally see—the tendency of professionals who work in the laboratory [to say]: "Oh, no, it's no big deal. It doesn't hurt. The ear is [just] cartilage. It's not going to hurt at all, etc. etc." But in practice, I think it's different because people complain a lot. Some leave really nervous with unpleasant reactions. . . . I think sometimes people exaggerate with the collection of material [samples] so that everyone can see how it's done or how it's not done. So my question is in this vein: Is it that this collection [of the skin smear] and the biopsy is just for the

education of these students or is it really important or necessary
for these patients?

She said that she has seen cases in which people no longer want to be
treated at the clinic after going through these diagnostic procedures
without proper orientation. While these procedures often may be
deemed medically necessary, providing patients with information on
what they might expect from them might go a long way to ensure that
patients follow through with treatment.

Another technique for diagnosis and determination of the extent
of nerve damage is the use of sensitivity tests, using either plastic filaments of different width and hardness or cotton balls dipped in hot and
cold liquid. These are not generally painful, but it is important for physicians to communicate with patients what they are trying to discover.
I have witnessed at least three sensitivity tests in which the patient was
either confused by the procedure or too nervous to properly comply.
For example, in a sensitivity test conducted by a male physical therapist using filaments of different strength, a female patient was asked to
close her eyes and say "*Senti*" ("I felt it") every time she felt something.
She began to say, "Senti, senti, senti," in quick succession, not always
corresponding to a touch with the filament. After a moment or two, the
physical therapist stopped and sat back. The woman, with eyes closed
and nothing being done to her, continued to say, "Senti, senti, senti."
He told her to open her eyes and informed her kindly that he had not
touched her with the filament. She protested that she had indeed felt
something, but admitted that she was also extremely nervous. We all
laughed about it, and the test was resumed after she took a few deep
breaths and concentrated on the test.

In this case, it was fortunate that the physical therapist was sensitive to the needs of the patient and realized that, unconsciously or con-
sciously, she was providing erroneous information about her sensitivity
during the test. It seemed that she was, on one hand, making a con-
certed effort to give the doctor the information she thought he wanted
to hear. On the other hand, with eyes closed and quite nervous, she may
also have believed she was feeling something. The filaments produce
little more sensation than a light tap from the tooth of a comb or the

fiber from a toothbrush. I observed several patients who had a hard time understanding at first what they were supposed to be doing during the hot and cold sensitivity test. Some patients would keep their eyes open and simply say "hot" or "cold," based on which hand the doctor was using. Generally, however, if provided with a simple explanation of for the purpose of the test, the patient might better understand what was expected and why it was necessary that the response be accurate.

Talking about Illness

Patients learn what disease they have, from a biomedical perspective, in different ways. As public health-related educational campaigns have increased, some people, including two patients I interviewed, diagnose themselves. When I conducted my research, referral to specialized treatment centers for hanseníase often gave away the potential diagnosis before the patients arrived, although not all patients knew what hanseníase was or that it might be a synonym for lepra. Some, who come to these clinics without knowledge of what they might have, learn that they have been sent to a leprosy or Hansen's disease treatment center from other patients they talk to while they await their first appointment. Others first hear the name of their disease from a health-care worker (often a social worker). The initial conversation with medical or social service staff that includes not only the name of the disease but also a discussion of a treatment regimen and the disease prognosis, is extremely important in shaping patients' explanatory models of their illness. Patients compare what they learn in this initial meeting with their personal experience of leprosy.

From my observations and interviews with patients, I noticed that certain forms of information were withheld from patients during this initial explanation of illness. As mentioned in chapter 3, some health-care workers make a point to avoid use of the term *lepra*, so that the patient does not self-stigmatize. In my observations, physicians and nurses did not always warn patients of the potential side effects of medications, assuming that patients either would not take the medications or that knowledge of these side effects would induce a psychosomatic response. The possibility of leprosy reaction, which occurs in

25–30 percent of people affected by leprosy, is also rarely brought up unless a patient is already in reaction at the time of diagnosis. Instead, patients are told to come in to the clinic if they experienced "anything unusual." Jessica Gregg (2003), who conducted ethnographic research with women with cervical cancer in Recife, Brazil, found a similar trend among physicians there, who typically withheld information about a patient's prognosis and the side effects of radiation therapy.

In part, these different examples of how authoritative knowledge is managed by healthcare professionals in Brazil may be an extension of the pre-existing paternalistic relationship with patients. Healthcare workers make decisions about what is best for patients, who, it is sometimes assumed, would not be able to process certain types of information because of their education or social class. They may be wary of scaring patients away by overloading them with worst-case scenarios of their illness. Another argument against disclosing too much information about leprosy upon a patient's first visit is that the patient might experience the well-documented nocebo phenomenon (the converse of the better-known placebo effect) in which negative symptoms are induced through suggestion (Hahn 1998), as when one reads the potential side-effects label too closely on one's prescription medication and begins to experience symptoms that perhaps would not otherwise have developed. However, if patients do have problems related to medication side effects or leprosy reaction, they may shift their explanatory models about leprosy's curability and distrust what they have learned from healthcare professionals. They may become frustrated, depressed, and even skeptical of the possibility of a cure. I believe that it is important for healthcare workers to find a middle ground between overwhelming patients with information that might unnecessarily frighten them and withholding all information about what they might expect with their treatment and illness.

Treating the Disease

Administering treatment is another important arena of interaction between doctors and patients. The World Health Organization (WHO) has set the standards for how treatment is to be administered in Brazil.

Rather than receive a supply of medications to last throughout their treatment, patients must come into a health post on a monthly basis to receive a supervised dose of medication of rifampicin plus, for multibacillary patients, clofazimine. The concept of the supervised dose at the clinic indicates an element of distrust in the ability of patients to care for themselves. However, it is meant as a way to regularly check on the patient, to follow up with their care, and to make sure no disabilities have been incurred. Patients are given a month's supply of MDT medications to take home for daily self-administration (clofazimine and dapsone for multibacillary patients and dapsone alone for paucibacillary patients). At their clinic visits, patients are expected to take a once-monthly dose of rifampicin in the presence of a nurse or doctor.

Giving instructions for taking the medicines at home can be problematic if the healthcare workers do not take the patient's life circumstances into account. Artur Custódio de Sousa of MORHAN uses the example of a patient who is told she must take the medications with a glass of milk every day. If the patient cannot afford milk, she, attempting to be as compliant as possible with medical instructions, decides not to take the medication at all since she cannot take it as instructed. In this example, the healthcare worker takes it for granted that the patient has milk available on a daily basis, or, alternatively, that the patient will understand that taking the medicine is more important than the drink with which it is taken. Milk is recommended to prevent stomach discomfort, but other liquids may be used as well. This misunderstanding could be avoided if healthcare workers instructed patients to take their medicine even if they cannot take it with milk.

In another example in which life circumstances of patients are not considered, physicians often tell patients with advanced cases of leprosy they can wash their eyes out with water to protect them and keep them free from particles. I have heard healthcare workers tell patients to drink a lot of water also, in order to keep their skin well hydrated. However, some patients live in areas where the water is not clean and could possibly be a source of further health problems. I believe that in these examples, healthcare workers take for granted that patients will have access to clean water for drinking and rinsing out their eyes. A better solution for the eyes would be to provide an eyewash solution, as some leprosy clinics do, and to instruct patients on ways to purify their water supply for washing and drinking. There are also other methods for hydrating the skin, including the use of Vaseline, which was sometimes provided to patients in small amounts to take home. Healthcare workers need to consider the daily lives of patients and how their situation will affect their treatment. Ideally, medical education could incorporate cultural and socioeconomic information that would give healthcare workers a better understanding of the circumstances of the patients from low-income communities.

Medication Side Effects

The side effects of the medications used for MDT and for leprosy reaction are numerous and made the experience of leprosy treatment extremely difficult for many of the patients with whom I spoke. Of the forty-three individuals I interviewed, two had not yet received their diagnosis and one had begun treatment on the day of the interview. The remaining forty patients were taking or had taken MDT and, in some cases, drugs for leprosy reaction such as prednisone or thalidomide. Of these forty, twenty-nine suffered side effects from the medications. Drug reactions are not the same as "leprosy reaction," the latter being the host's reaction to leprosy bacilli, described in more detail in chapter 1. However, I was not always sure if the "reactions" patients described were from the medications or from leprosy reaction, and patients were not always clear about the difference. I have tried to make a distinction between the problems patients described that would be classified biomedically as side effects of medications and those that are part of the disease process (leprosy symptoms, for example, or problems associated with leprosy reaction).

Dapsone can cause severe allergies, gastritis, headache, and anemia, among other effects. Isabela Maria Bernades Goulart et al. (2002), in a study of 187 leprosy patients in the state of Minas Gerais in Brazil, found that dapsone was responsible for the majority (70.7 percent) of the reported side effects of MDT in some patients. Only one patient (Patrícia, twenty-two) in my sample mentioned specifically having a reaction to dapsone, but many patients did not know this drug by name but rather recognized it as a "little white pill," most likely because the medication names are not written on the blister packs of pills. Since patients on MDT were taking two or three medications at once, they were not always aware of which MDT drugs were causing side effects. With the combined difficulties of everyday life and of having leprosy, it was also difficult to differentiate medication side effects from symptoms that may result from other forms of stress. Humberto, age fifty, said that when he began MDT, he had bad headaches, but he was not sure "whether it was from the medicine or just from something in general." I talked to several patients who complained of headaches, which are possible side effects of both dapsone and rifampicin. Milene, a little girl in treatment for leprosy who was featured on a Discovery Channel documentary (Ward 1999) in which I participated, had been treated at a health post in Rio and had a severe reaction to dapsone. I asked her mother about this in the interview I conducted for that documentary:

MOTHER: Yes, she had a reaction, was in the hospital for ten days because the medication made her ill. Then she stopped taking the medication. Now, they're treating her but without this medication . . .

C.W.: Were you very worried?

MOTHER: She was all purple, sort of purple. I thought she was going to die. Her mouth was purple, her tongue was purple. Her hands and feet, all purple. We got to the hospital and they said they didn't have the medicine they needed to give her. She was on serum [an i.v.] for three days, just with serum, nothing else, and she got better little by little.

This reaction may have been an allergic reaction or the result of a healthcare worker accidentally administering an adult dosage of dapsone to her.

The drug clofazimine causes the skin to dry out, creating a scaly effect known as ichthyosis (from the Greek word for "fish," *icthys*). This drying may be responsible for the itching that several patients experienced. Leprosy does not, according to the biomedical model, cause itching, but some patients insisted that "their illness" was very itchy. Another common side effect of clofazimine is a change in skin color, sometimes giving it an almost bluish or reddish tint, but primarily darkening it, often unevenly. This effect is more noticeable in people with lighter skin.

In an oral history I transcribed from Carville (that was conducted by Julia Elwood), former resident José Ramirez, Jr. recounted how clofazimine-related skin changes affected him in early 1970s Louisiana. Mr. Ramirez, who now resides in Houston, Texas, and serves as a coordinator for IDEA (International Association for "Integration Dignity and Economic Advancement"), an international NGO that works to eliminate leprosy stigma, gave me permission to use his name and to include the following excerpt from his life history:

> I was put on what is known as B663. It's got a technical name for
> it that I don't recall right now. That particular medication serves
> as a dye, and it focuses on the areas where the bacilli is located.
> But it also turns the complexion of the skin very dark. For some
> patients, it focuses only on the areas where the bacilli is found.
> For others, it just affects the whole area. With me, I turned so
> black, or dark that, it's ironic—when I was going to school at LSU
> [Louisiana State University], at the end of the registration line is
> where you have all the student organizations. All the foreign stu-
> dent associations were trying to get me to sign up because they
> thought I looked foreign, like an Indian from India. Then when
> I started teaching at Southern [University, in Baton Rouge], and
> I would walk by people for whatever reason, I was called, "Hey
> brother." That changed very rapidly as soon as they heard my
> alleged accent. . . . That was a little traumatic for me because
> when I would go [home], people would look at me in a state of
> shock, as if, "What the heck is going on? What is happening to
> your body? What is happening to your skin?"
>
> It also had some negative effects for me personally because
> I remember one time in particular when [my girlfriend] and
> I—she had come down to visit—and we had decided to go to
> New Orleans for the day. We were walking around in the French
> Quarter, and there was this guy in back of us that said, "What is
> that white bitch doing with that nigger?" And I was able to under-
> stand the fear that a black person feels when that happens. Of

course, being brown originally myself, I had experienced some of
that discrimination as well, but it put a lot of fear in both—not
only me, but also in [my girlfriend].

I also experienced—when my skin was very dark and we were
driving back to Laredo for a visit, and we decided to stop in Breaux
Bridge to get some crawfish, and in order to get to Breaux Bridge
or to a restaurant called Ferguson's, you had to get off the main
road and go down a little road. It has what I considered a speed
trap, 'cause it has a very small sign that says thirty miles per hour
and I was going forty. I got stopped by this policeman who came
out, had his hands on his gun, and kept calling me "boy." He kept
asking how come a "nigger boy" could have [a Latino surname].
He could not understand. At the time, [we] were just wondering
what was going on. Eventually, he had me write out the ticket
because I found out that he was illiterate. He couldn't write, but
he kept calling me "boy" and [telling me] how ignorant I was and
then forced me to drive down to the police station, and I paid the
ticket. He said he was not going to issue a ticket, he was going
to have me sign out the ticket and pay for it. So it has some con-
notations that made me get closer to Louisiana and to Louisiana
blacks in particular because of the discoloration of my skin.

Although none of the people I interviewed in Brazil mentioned
experiencing specific incidents of racial discrimination, several were
frustrated both by the alteration in their appearance and by the con-
stant questioning by friends and relatives. Afonso, fifty, reported that
several of his friends commented on the change in his skin color.
According to Afonso, they told him, "'You're turning black [*preto*].
What's that?' I'm taking the medicines and this is what's happening. . . .
Everyone was worried because of this medicine . . . People asked, 'How
is this medicine making you darker [*mais moreno*]?' I don't want to take
this medicine anymore." Cláudio, twenty-one, was taking clofazimine at
the time of the interview and said, "I'm having this now, that I'm darker
[*mais escuro*]. He [the doctor] said that it had to be like this. [It's like]
tanning lotion [*bronzeador*]." Although the doctor tried to put a positive
spin on this change in skin color, darker skin is associated with lower

status in Brazil, and a change in skin color could potentially have negative consequences.

Rifampicin, which is taken only once a month by patients, often causes side effects in the first few days after administration. A large dose, 600 mg, is given to both multibacillary and paucibacillary patients when they come to the clinic for a new blister pack. According to the Brazilian Ministry of Health, "loss of appetite, nausea, occasionally vomit and diarrhea, and light abdominal pain" can occur with rifampicin. "These symptoms will probably occur if the medication is ingested on an empty stomach" (Ministério de Saúde 1994, 93), yet it is still recommended to take it this way for maximum effectiveness. Wilson, thirty-six, had just begun treatment at the time I interviewed him and described side effects that may have been from rifampicin: "I felt very bad. I think it's because of the side effects. I had fever. I still get a fever when I use a lot of energy. But now I seem to be getting used to it. In the first week, I also vomited. I was nauseous. Lots of chills. But now it's o.k."

Other side effects of rifampicin have to do with its properties as an antibiotic. Antibiotics reduce the effectiveness of birth control pills and cause greater sensitivity to the sun. Although I heard physicians warn patients about sun sensitivity, I did not on any occasion hear a physician warn a female patient about the possibility that birth control pills could fail while on rifampicin. One physician was giving a first-time patient orientation about her disease. The physician turned to me and asked me if I thought she was leaving anything out. I asked the patient if she was on birth control; she was, so I told her that she might have to use a back-up method. The doctor said she always forgot to mention that, but that it was very important. This lack of warning about the different possible consequences of antibiotics is not unique to leprosy treatment of course, nor to Brazil, perhaps because antibiotics are so commonly prescribed. Even if the possibility of pregnancy is slight, patients should be given the opportunity to take steps to prevent it, particularly while they are in treatment for leprosy. Before a law was passed controlling thalidomide distribution, this drug was being prescribed to women who were also taking rifampicin, so even if they were taking birth control pills, they could get pregnant, thus increasing the likelihood of having babies born with thalidomide syndrome.

Medications for leprosy reactions seemed to create the most problematic side effects for the patients I interviewed. The steroid prednisone is a drug that often causes a physiological dependency, so that the
dosage must be gradually reduced or the patient's reaction will return
stronger than before. For leprosy reaction, physicians are supposed to
start patients on sixty milligrams of prednisone a day for patients who
weigh close to sixty kilograms. The dosage is then gradually reduced by
ten milligrams a week, or as the patient improves (Ministério de Saúde
1994). Patients often become frustrated because as soon as they reach
lower dosages, they experience problems and the doctors return them
to a higher dosage, from which they have to come down slowly. Zé, fifty-
five, described his situation on prednisone: "It's always like that. Always
when I stop taking the medicine and I'm discharged, one month later I
start to feel bad."

Patrícia, twenty-two, was on twenty milligrams of prednisone at the
time of my interview with her, but she had been hospitalized for leprosy
reactions in the past, and she was taking up to one hundred milligrams
a day at one point:

> I started taking prednisone halfway through the treatment
> [MDT]. Then I stopped . . . but then I had nerve problems in my
> hand, I was sad and in pain. Then I had to take a higher dose.
> I kept taking it and taking it and taking it, but when I reached
> fifty milligrams, I was all pocked [*pipocada*]—edemas, as they say,
> edemas . . . now they're giving me azathioprine and pentoxifyl-
> line, but pentox is giving me stomach pains. Now I'm taking a
> lot. I hope they take me off these soon . . . because I'm taking
> too much.

Aside from physical dependency, prednisone, a steroid, causes rapid
weight gain and facial swelling. This change in appearance caused by
prolonged use of prednisone was particularly traumatic for many of the
women I interviewed. Patrícia said, "I had such a complex, not even
because of the disease [but because of] this fat—I gained a lot of weight.
He [the doctor] said that with prednisone, you retain liquids, right?" For
Patrícia, who said she was very thin before, this weight gain was very
stressful. In urban Brazil, a slender body is the ideal for women across

socioeconomic strata. The changes in her appearance brought on by prednisone lowered her self-esteem, made her more withdrawn, and caused her to eat more:

> My body changed a lot. So I don't have—my wardrobe, all my pretty clothes are put away. They don't fit me. So I gave my bikini away because I had to buy a larger one for myself. . . . [Eventually] I stopped going to the beach.

Prednisone also causes stomach problems, including gastritis and even peptic ulcers (Ministério de Saúde 1994, 95). Many patients I observed were given ranitidine to take with prednisone. Ranitidine is the primary ingredient in many medications used to control stomach acid. Leprosy patients taking prednisone were taking 150 milligrams of ranitidine per dose, twice the recommended dosage of the North American over-the-counter medication Zantac, for example. Zé, fifty-five, said that he always has stomach problems: "This is my great affliction . . . I take ranitidine to combat this stomach pain." Gerson, twenty-three, in discussing his medications, told me that he was also taking ranitidine for his stomach problems because, as he said, "it affects the stomach, prednisone. Ah, I'm feeling a lot of stomach pain, that burning." Manoel, thirty, complained that prednisone caused nausea and loss of appetite.

Thalidomide is an alternative to prednisone in terms of its effectiveness in treating leprosy reactions without many side effects. However, as mentioned in chapter 1, thalidomide causes serious birth defects in children of mothers who take the drug during a certain period of their pregnancy. Thalidomide is one of the best drugs available for leprosy reaction, but many women are excluded from this drug today because of the nature of thalidomide and the inability, in Brazil, to provide the proper assurances that a woman of reproductive age who is taking the drug will not get pregnant. It is still distributed to men, thus presenting the risk of drug sharing. In 1995, during preliminary research, I watched as a medical intern shouted instructions to an elderly man who was very hard of hearing on how and when to take the thalidomide she was giving him to take home, telling him to make sure his daughter assisted him. I was concerned that he may not have understood or heard the instructions and that the thalidomide he was taking home could fall into anyone's hands. After nearly ten years of thinking about the thalidomide issue in leprosy treatment, I do not think that thalidomide should be banned for distribution to patients for whom this drug would be beneficial in controlling leprosy reaction, but I do feel that measures should be taken to ensure that more babies with thalidomide syndrome are not being born. Artur Custódio de Sousa of MORHAN uses the following analogy to discuss the risks and benefits of thalidomide: Thousands of people die or are disabled each year on the highways, yet we do not ban cars. Instead, there is an attempt to ensure that protections are in place to minimize danger, with mechanisms such as safety standards for cars, speed limits, and seat belt laws. In the United States, thalidomide has been approved for use in leprosy, AIDS, and cancer treatments for men and women, but women of reproductive age are required to take frequent pregnancy tests.

Aside from the teratogenic, or birth-defect-causing effect of thalidomide, there are other side effects. Because it is also a powerful sedative, thalidomide makes patients very sleepy, and it must be taken at night for this reason. Patients sometimes reported impotence as another side effect. Zé, fifty-five, said that he suffered from impotence, which he believed was a result of the medications, although he did not say specifically that he was taking thalidomide. Xavier, thirty-two, who was on 300 milligrams of thalidomide per day (the standard dose for patients in reaction can be anywhere from 100–400 milligrams), told me that thalidomide and the other medicines have greatly affected his sex life:

> It's a joke. Any [desire] I had is gone. [The doctor] said that it's all
> in my head. It sure isn't. . . . It's not just this one [thalidomide].
> All of the medicines diminished [my sexual desire]—40 percent
> of my potency went away.

The side effects of medications are a potential motivation for abandonment of treatment. For some patients, the negative prospect of taking medicines for a long period of time keeps patients from seeking treatment in the first place. Alícia, thirty-nine, who had never abandoned treatment herself, told me that her sister-in-law had leprosy but was not in treatment because she was "afraid" of it. The primary solutions to this problem would be to reduce the duration of treatment, a strategy that is currently being tested, and to improve the selection and quality of drugs available for leprosy reaction. Healthcare workers can also explain to patients that most side effects, such as the change in skin tone with clofazimine, are temporary. One volunteer I interviewed said that if patients know what to expect in terms of side effects, they are more likely to adhere to treatment if these side effects appear. Patients, she said, stop taking medications because they make them feel worse than they did before they began the treatment and because "the doctor never explained that this was [a normal] reaction to the medication."

Interpretations of Leprosy Reaction

At the beginning of treatment, the first question people ask is usually: "Does this have a cure?" Wilson, twenty-eight, who had recently begun treatment when I interviewed him, expressed this concern:

> Even now I'm always worried about whether or not I'm going to be cured. That's what anyone would think about. If anything appears [anything like a symptom], you get worried. "Will this really go o.k., will I really be o.k., soon?"

The answer that patients receive from healthcare professionals to the question of whether leprosy is curable is an emphatic "yes." However, the reality for some patients seems very different. Although patients who complete the WHO-recommended MDT treatment program are declared *alta* (discharged) and *curado* (cured), many patients continue to have leprosy reactions for several years after the designation of "alta" is given. Some patients are left with extensive nerve damage and physical deformity. These patients may not accept that they are cured because in the case of reaction, they are experiencing symptoms that are just as bad as or worse than before they began treatment. The idea that all of the bacilli are killed is meaningless if they continue to feel ill. Likewise, for patients who have become disabled due to leprosy, they will continue to suffer affliction from the disease for the rest of their lives, and thus they may still consider themselves to be sick (*doente*).

Leprosy reaction can be very confusing for patients since they often see new lesions appear in the same spots where they had them in the past. They may experience more physical discomfort that they did from the symptoms of leprosy itself. Many patients misunderstand what is happening to their bodies and believe they are having a reaction to the medications. This is reinforced by healthcare professionals who use the term "reaction" (reação). Also, because leprosy reaction is common shortly after patients begin MDT, patients assume this condition is an indication that the treatment is making them worse.

Fernando, twenty, had a major reaction almost in the same month in which he finished his MDT and was told he was "alta": Then, he said, "my ear was infiltrated [with bacilli], the sores emerged, all in less than a week. My foot was swollen . . . and [I was] in pain. . . . An incredible pain. I've never felt so much pain." Such a reaction at the end of treatment is confusing and frustrating for patients who had hoped to be finished with the disease and treatment when they took their last dose of MDT. Renata, thirty-six, who had her first symptoms in 1988, continued to suffer from reaction when I interviewed her (in 1998) and did not believe there was a cure for her:

> I don't believe in it. I could wind up changing my opinion. The day I'm feeling good, I'll believe it. The day I don't feel anything [pain], then o.k. But as long as I'm feeling something, the illness is not over. The day that I'm o.k., I'll even put it in the newspaper!

Andrade (1997) noted the difference between biomedical and patient definitions of being "cured" of leprosy after a patient told her that he did not "feel cured," despite being told by doctors he was cured. The difference in the meaning of the word "cure" for doctors and patients was significant in terms of how patients felt and behaved. This was true among patients I interviewed as well. Patients expressed frustration with physicians for telling them they were cured when obviously, to them, they were still sick. Patients equated physical discomfort and disability with disease. Being "cured" is synonymous with a return to health, to "normal" body functioning, or regular body functioning as defined by them. These definitions of disease and cure are certainly not limited to patient explanatory models but are close to the standard, accepted definitions for these concepts. For example, *Webster's New World Dictionary* defines *cure* as "restoration to health or a sound condition" (Neufeldt and Guralink 1988, 339). Yet under the current MDT treatment program, patients are said to be "cured" after treatment is complete, whether or not they have experienced a complete "restoration to health." To meet the goal of treating existing patients so as to halt the transmission of leprosy worldwide, the WHO definition of cure is adequate. However, for patients who continue to experience leprosy-related problems after MDT is complete, the concept of "cure" should encompass treatment for leprosy reaction as well.

The idea of leprosy as curable is important in reducing stigma associated with the disease. At the same time, when healthcare workers present information to patients about their disease at diagnosis, I think it is important to let patients know about the possibility of leprosy reaction taking place. In addition, rather than argue with patients (as I have observed healthcare workers doing), telling them that they are "cured" and no longer have leprosy, even though they are still experiencing symptoms that are related to the disease, healthcare workers should perhaps find a way to acknowledge patients' suffering while helping them understand the process of treatment for leprosy reaction.

I observed or learned about a few interesting metaphors employed by healthcare workers to explain leprosy reaction to patients once it occurred. Some physicians and nurses use a version of the following metaphor to explain leprosy reactions to patients. (I heard this used on one occasion by a nurse, and a volunteer said she also used this metaphor to explain reactions):

> When you spray insecticide for roaches, it kills the roaches, but then you have many dead roach bodies lying around. You are not going to leave them there. You sweep them up. Likewise, your body has dead bacilli that have been killed by the multidrug therapy, but your body still has a cleaning job to do.

With this analogy, healthcare workers are trying to convey the message that once the MDT is complete, the patient is cured, but the body still has to rid itself of bacilli, which can produce new symptoms. Some healthcare workers use a military metaphor to help patients understand reactions. I discovered that this metaphor was in use during a workshop on leprosy education at MORHAN, where volunteers brought it up as the way in which they explained reaction. This metaphor posits the patient's body as a battlefield, with the bacilli being enemy soldiers. At the end of the battle, there are dead soldiers and their body parts lying all around the battlefield. Something must be done to get rid of this debris. The broken soldiers' bodies and body parts represent the broken bacilli. Emily Martin (1994) noted that the use of military metaphors in biomedical discourse is a product of the increasing militarism worldwide in the twentieth century. The media has played a large role in perpetuating the idea of the body as a fortress to be defended and of viruses and bacteria as foreign invaders. Though a bit grim, I think both of these metaphors could be effective tools for explaining the process of leprosy reaction to patients. These explanations might be employed at diagnosis, however, rather than at the first occurrence of leprosy reaction, so that patients will understand that leprosy reaction, if they experience it, is neither a reaction to the medications nor a sign that their medications are not working.

Abandonment of Treatment

Adherence to the medications of MDT for leprosy is important for several reasons. Patients who abandon the treatment program before it is complete may have a relapse of the disease and may continue transmitting the disease to others. In addition, patients who cease taking their medications and who stop coming into the health post run the risk of developing severe disabilities. Leprosy patients confront many problems related to the treatment and their illness that might lead to abandonment. Some of these problems have been discussed in this chapter so far—problems with the medical system, communication problems with healthcare workers, side effects of treatment, and so on. Certain problems exist for many patients but might provoke one patient to abandon treatment whereas others persist.

The average abandonment rates for MDT treatment between 1994 and 1997 in Rio de Janeiro (the years just before I began my research)

were 5.3 percent for paucibacillary patients and 10.1 percent for multibacillary patients (Gerência de Dermatologia Sanitária 1998). Most
of my formal interviews with patients were conducted at a health
post with a relatively higher rate of adherence. Since the patients I
met were complying with the treatment, I was unable to collect much
data from these interviews about reasons for abandonment, although
there were a few patients who had abandoned treatment temporarily
or who had irregular attendance at the clinic. I did, however, learn
more about reasons for abandonment from interviews with healthcare
workers and volunteers at MORHAN, who answered the "Telehansen"
lines, presented puppet shows to schoolchildren, and occasionally
made house visits to patients who had abandoned treatment. According to volunteers, unanticipated side effects of treatment were a major
reason for abandonment.

In a study of leprosy patients in Rio de Janeiro, Claro (1995, 75)
found that patients' reasons for temporary abandonment of treatment
or missed appointments included: "the occurrence of strikes among
health professionals, taking trips, denial of the illness, the occurrence
of reactional episodes, undesirable effects of the medicine, and lack of
information about clinical aspects of the disease." In her study of how
leprosy affects men and women in Riberão Preto, São Paulo, Maria Hel-
ena de Oliveira found that men and women have different reasons for
abandoning treatment or for irregular attendance at the health post.
Using a structured questionnaire with 202 leprosy patients (132 men
and 70 women), her results were as follows:

> With respect to compliance to the treatment and clinic atten-
> dance, seventy percent of women and sixty percent of men
> complied with treatment. Forgotten appointments, undesirable
> side-effects, fear of medication, preference for alcoholic bever-
> ages, loss of work, and disbelief in the diagnosis were the reasons
> men gave for their absences. Women mentioned adverse reac-
> tions to treatment as the main impediment, followed by forget-
> fulness. (Oliveira 1997, 3)

Alcoholic beverages are not supposed to be consumed during treatment
because they make the MDT medications less effective and because

both alcohol and the medications affect the liver. In Rio de Janeiro, drinking beer or liquor is an important part of daily life and of masculine identity, and it may be a factor in some cases of nonadherence to treatment. Four patients, all men, mentioned drinking as something they had to reluctantly curtail because of MDT, though this restriction did not prevent them from complying with treatment.

On a brief trip to Manaus in 1999, I interviewed a nurse and representative of the Instituto Alfredo da Matta, where they treat patients from all over Amazonas state for leprosy, tuberculosis, AIDS, and other infectious diseases. I asked her what she thought the reasons for abandonment of treatment were in the Amazon, and she said that disbelief in the cure was the number one reason. Sônia, forty-four, who suffered leprosy reaction for years after her treatment ended and worked as a volunteer for MORHAN in Rio de Janeiro occasionally, said she has met many patients who have abandoned their treatment, and she also said the primary reason given was not believing that there was a cure for their illness. When patients do not feel like they are getting better, there is no motivation for continuing treatment.

Of the forty patients I interviewed who already had begun treatment, only one claimed to have abandoned it for a length of time that required starting it over from the beginning upon returning to the clinic. Eight patients I interviewed had missed an appointment or missed a few days of medicine at some point. Irregular attendance is not the same as complete abandonment of treatment, but it can have negative effects on the patient's treatment program. These patients missed appointments for reasons related to work, family problems, other illnesses, and transportation. Some patients missed appointments because they could not pay for transportation to a clinic or health post, which is discussed in more detail below.

Gerson, twenty-three, was the one patient who abandoned treatment for several months because of a trip to Bahia, the state where he was born: "I went to Bahia. So I abandoned [treatment]. Then I had to start all over again when I returned from Bahia. Because this is no joke . . . if you're going to get better, you have to take the medications correctly." Because clinics give out only one blister pack a month, patients may not know they can request more packs for a special occasion or a trip, and some physicians may not comply with this request. One aspect of leprosy treatment that is problematic is that patients are expected to stick with one doctor or clinic throughout their treatment. From a medical point of view, this makes sense because each case of leprosy is different, and it is useful for doctors to monitor a patient's progress with medications and history of reactions or other complications. However, because treatment lasts for several months, it is impractical to assume that all patients will remain in the same location throughout treatment. Some patients move to a different city or state during treatment, either temporarily or permanently, for work or other reasons. A MORHAN volunteer said that some of the patients he works with are truck drivers, who are out of town for long periods of time. Through government legislation, MORHAN was trying to make it easier for patients to go to health posts in different cities to be treated at any stage during their treatment, without having to go through the diagnostic exams again or start treatment from the beginning.

Many patients who miss appointments or stop taking medication temporarily do so because of circumstances beyond their control. For example, Fernando, twenty, simply forgot to bring his medications along on a trip: "I think I went only five days without [the medications] in the woods. I went camping, and I forgot the medications in the other bag of medicines." Cláudio, twenty-one, said that he missed one appointment because he had an emergency with his son. Denise, twenty-seven, underwent a severe reaction, for which she was supposed to see the doctor, but she was having bad back problems (unrelated to leprosy) and could not make it to the clinic.

None of the patients I interviewed deliberately abandoned treatment because of problems or frustrations with either the treatment or the medical services available to them. Many had these problems, but for them, it was not motivation enough to abandon treatment altogether. The irregular attendance of some patients usually had to do with practicalities of their daily lives. Again, a good adherence rate may have to do with the fact that the clinic where I conducted interviews did not run out of medications and has a well-equipped facility with several caring doctors, nurses, and a social worker. Of course, my sample of patients is somewhat biased because I interviewed the patients who were receiving treatment at the clinic; none had permanently abandoned treatment.

In a 1997 document, WHO recommended that the following steps be taken regarding abandonment of treatment:

> a) the centre should review the treatment register annually during the month of January; b) prepare a list of patients who did not collect treatment during the last twelve months; c) visit homes of such patients during the month of January and persuade them to return for assessment and, if necessary, continuation of treatment; d) if a patient is not available during the first visit, request family or friends or neighbors to persuade the patient to report to the centre; e) if the patient does not report within a week, make a second visit to his/her home; f) by the end of January, review the treatment register and remove defaulters who are unlikely to come back; g) if any defaulter returns subsequently, make a careful clinical examination (with skin smears, if available) and if found to have signs of active leprosy, re-register and start a new course of appropriate MDT regimen. (WHO 1997)

In an attempt to "rescue" or "recapture" (*resgatar*) patients who have abandoned treatment, some clinics in Rio de Janeiro have social workers or others make house visits to patients to talk to them and find out why they abandoned treatment. MORHAN volunteers worked closely with the health post in Nova Iguaçu and made these house visits to patients who had abandoned treatment there, but for the eleven months I was in Brazil, MORHAN's office and the health post there were *em obras* (under construction), so this service was put on hold. In addition, MORHAN had only one car available for this type of visit. I was able to make house visits with a social worker from one outpatient treatment center where I attended educational waiting-room meetings. She had occasional access to the ambulance that was used to transport residents of a former leprosarium to the city for medical services not available on the grounds and to transport the bodies of residents who had passed away to a funeral home or cemetery. I was able to accompany the social worker on house visits on two occasions.

Both attempts to make house visits were relatively futile. Each time we drove around for several hours in the municipality of Jacarepaguá and adjacent areas. Much of the time was spent in pursuit of addresses. We attempted to contact a total of seven patients who had abandoned treatment. At two addresses, no one was home, but after leaving a note at one of the addresses, we found out later that the patient had died. We were unable to locate one address. At another, we were told that the patient had moved and left no forwarding address. Two other patients had moved but a relative at the address said they would relay the clinic's phone number to them. One patient was at work, and we spoke to his father. Thus we were unable to contact any of the patients directly.

Although house visits could be useful in getting some patients to return to the clinic, most health posts do not have the resources to support this type of activity. The social worker at one health post in a suburb of Rio told me she wanted to visit some patients who had abandoned treatment, but she was required to use her own car and save gas receipts to be reimbursed later. She had so many duties at the health post, it was difficult to find time to make house visits. In addition, many of the patients live in favelas that are controlled by drug traffickers and that are not easily accessible to nonresidents. MORHAN volunteers told me of a visit they made to a favela to attempt to locate a patient who had abandoned treatment. Men armed with machine guns stopped them at the entrance to the favela, but when they explained why they were there, one of the armed men said the patient was his brother, and he accompanied them to his house. They said the man threatened his brother and said he would make sure he complied with the treatment from then on. Although this house visit was "successful," there is a certain amount of risk involved in making these visits because of the presence of drug trafficking and of an insider-outsider dichotomy in many favelas.

House visits can also be somewhat invasive. When searching for an address, the social worker I accompanied on house visits never said that the person she was looking for was being treated for hanseníase, but she did mention that she worked at a facility that was formerly a leprosarium. In addition, we made house visits in an ambulance, which might have aroused suspicion among the neighbors and created problems for patients who had perhaps not revealed to neighbors or even family members that they had an illness.

Although different nations have their own policies for determining rates of abandonment, WHO sets the standards for determining if a patient has abandoned treatment: "A defaulter is a person who has not collected treatment for twelve consecutive months" (WHO 2003, 97). A true picture of the number of patients who have abandoned treatment and not returned is not possible, because these "defaulters" are no longer counted in the statistics after a certain period of time. WHO encourages follow-up of patients, but, as outlined in the "Defaulter Management Action" plan quoted above, patients who have not returned after twelve months and whom clinic representatives are not able to bring back are supposed to be taken off the patient registry (WHO 1997, 66). The problem with dropping patients from the record after a year is that clinics, and subsequently cities and nations, underestimate of the number of active cases of leprosy that exist.

Abandonment rates are based on the numbers or percentage of patients who stop taking MDT and do not return. However, there are other forms of abandoning treatment. There are no statistics on how many patients abandon their treatment for leprosy reaction or do not come in for scheduled follow-up appointments after MDT is complete. Many patients require medical care and reaction medications for years after they are technically "cured" of leprosy. Some patients tend not to be as vigilant after they receive the designation of "alta." Although most patients I interviewed were very good about making their appointments when they were on MDT, one said he missed follow-up appointments because his treatment was "complete" and he had been declared "alta." Vicente, twenty-eight, said that he never missed an appointment during his "treatment," but afterward, he would only come in when he was having a bad reaction and not on the scheduled appointment days.

Another form of abandoning treatment that is not measured in government or WHO statistics is adherence to physical therapy recommendations or sessions. These statistics are harder to come by because the availability of physical therapy services for patients is not universal. In interviews with thirty-three leprosy patients and their families in Campinas, Queiroz and Puntel (1997, 92) found that only about 15 percent of patients followed physical therapy recommendations for daily exercises. One physical therapist I observed, who worked at two different clinics I visited, often showed patients exercises they could do for their hands and gave them advice on soaking and bandaging their feet. Some of the advice is difficult to follow in the real world, where patients might not have the time for physical exercises or the resources to care for their feet, hands, and ulcers. Abandoning physical therapy or treatment for reactions is not monitored as closely because it does not contribute to disease transmission. However, these forms of abandoning treatment are just as harmful to the individual patient as abandonment of MDT and need to be taken into consideration if a true picture of leprosy's long-term effects on patients' lives is to be measured.

Logistics: Getting to the Clinic, Getting Treated

There are other issues related to the medical encounter that may be out of the hands of healthcare professionals but that affect patients' experience with leprosy treatment. For patients without their own car, getting to different zones of the city requires the use of one or more forms of public transportation. Taxis are common but are expensive for low-income Brazilians to afford on a regular basis. Rio has a good public bus system, and for most destinations, there are a number of city buses and routes that can get you where you want to go. On my most recent trip to Brazil in 2006, I noticed that many of the buses had been redesigned and more regular city buses were equipped with air conditioning. Rio also has a very modern subway system, but its route does not yet reach all parts of the city. Traveling between Rio de Janeiro and Niterói, which are on opposite sides of Guanabara Bay, requires a ferry ride. There is also a "light rail" train that extends to the suburbs of the Zona Norte. Still, time and money spent on transportation to a treatment center can be prohibitive for patients.

Because my research locations were spread out in different parts of the city, I spent many hours each week on every kind of public transportation available except for the train, and I had a chance to experience what getting to work and getting to the clinic might mean to the majority of working-class Brazilians. I gradually figured out the best routes to the places where I was working, but even then, traveling from my apartment to the health posts and to the offices of MORHAN required a minimum of an hour, often involving a bit of walking. To get to one outpatient treatment center I occasionally visited, two hours were generally required. There was a relatively expensive *frescão* (literally, ultra-cool, i.e., air-conditioned) bus that stopped in a plaza near our apartment and ran west along the beaches of the Zona Sul, but it came very infrequently. In order to attend educational waiting-room meetings, which began at eight in the morning, I chose a route with more frequent buses. I left the apartment in the dark, just before six o'clock, and took a bus to the Praça (Plaza) Mauá in downtown Rio. The bus was not crowded at that time; most passengers seemed to be on their way home after the night shift and slept through most of the ride. From the Praça Mauá, I took a bus along the edges of a large favela and over the mountains and slippery, steep roads of the rainforest-covered Serra dos Três Rios (Sierra of Three Rivers) to the municipality of Jacarepaguá.

In 1998 patients I interviewed were receiving public transportation vouchers (*vale-transporte*) provided by the government. I thought this was an excellent way to ensure patient adherence to treatment. However, in many cases, family members often accompanied patients to the health post for treatment. A twelve-year-old girl, awaiting a possible diagnosis of leprosy, came to the health post one day with her grandmother. They lived in Duque de Caxias, a municipality to the north of the clinic. The girl's grandmother complained that the clinic only provided bus vouchers for the girl and not for her.

By early 1999, I noticed that fewer patients received vouchers. I talked to clinic staff and found out that these were not provided on a regular basis by the government. Often they only had one-way passes to give to patients, and sometimes, none at all. Daniela, nineteen, lived in Campos Elíseos, a neighborhood in Duque de Caxias, outside Rio de Janeiro's city limits. Her bus fare from there to the clinic was R$2.50 each way, about U.S.$2.25 at the time of the interview. This fare was especially difficult for her to pay if she had to come to the clinic more than once a week, which had lately been the case, as she was undergoing severe episodes of leprosy reaction. Gerson, twenty-three, lived even farther away from the clinic:

I have to pay R$5.50 for the passage there and back. Sometimes you have this money. It's not every day that you have it though, right? So it's difficult sometimes. It's very far. But I like coming here. I don't want to go to the health post because here the treatment is much better. Here it's straightforward, easier.

Gerson made the decision to come to the clinic of his choice, even though the transportation costs were slightly higher, which is something Oliveira (1997) found to be common in her survey of leprosy patients in Ribeirão Preto, São Paulo. Of her sample of 202 patients, twenty-four percent came to Ribeirão Preto from other cities, primarily because they felt the quality of the treatment there was better than in the health facilities where they lived.

Renata, thirty-six, married with three children and unemployed at the time of the interview, said that to arrive at the clinic in the morning, she had to "leave home at dawn, and I can't be accompanied by my husband, because he works nights." She also had a problem with the cost of the trip, which was four reals:

I have to get buses and be on foot, full of pain. I have to stand [on the bus] from there to here. . . . It's two reals. A lot. That's one way. It's four reals [total]. They [the clinic] used to pay for [the passage] there and back. . . . The last time I came, they only gave me one way. That doesn't help.

Distance to a treatment center is a reason why some people do not seek treatment in the first place. Wilson, thirty-six, said his niece (his wife's brother's daughter) most likely has leprosy, but she had not been able to get to the hospital where she could be tested. His wife, who participated in the interview, said, "The hospital is very far from where she lives. . . . She's lost a lot of weight. She still hasn't started treatment, and it's been four years since this problem began."

The number of days in which health posts operate for leprosy treatment is a problem for some patients, especially those who work five to six days per week. The clinic where I conducted most of my research operated five days during the week for leprosy patients. They were open three days a week for eight-hour days and two half days, one of which was for families to come in for preventive vaccines. They were not open on weekends, which made it difficult for patients who worked during the week. Most health posts operated on a more restricted schedule for leprosy treatment, usually one or two half days a week with one physician in attendance. At a training session I attended on leprosy treatment held at MORHAN, a volunteer from Nova Iguaçu said the biggest problem for patients was missing work because of the limited hours that the clinic was open. He also said that in that municipality, six thousand leprosy patients were treated at one clinic with only four physicians and one nurse, which is why clinic hours were limited. A representative from the state health department who attended this session said that establishing Saturday clinics had been successful in many municipalities in Rio de Janeiro. Of course, incentives for physicians to attend Saturday clinics would need to be provided for this to be widely successful.

Lack of Medications

A large health problem often cited in Brazil is the lack of medications available in public health facilities. At public health clinics, medications are supposed to be provided by the government, but when supplies run out, patients must buy them from pharmacies or go without. On November 19, 1998, physicians and healthcare workers went on strike because of a lack of medications and basic supplies such as equipment to test for diabetes (Rede Globo Rio de Janeiro 1998). The newspaper *Jornal do Brasil* ran an investigation in July 1999 in which they found that half of the thirty-six health posts in the city of São Gonçalo (near Niterói in Rio de Janeiro state) had only two of the thirty types of medicines they were supposed to carry (*Jornal do Brasil* 1999).

Since 1991, MDT has been provided to patients free of charge by WHO, the pharmaceutical company Novartis, and the Japanese Nippon Foundation (or Sasakawa Foundation); there should always be an adequate supply of MDT blister-packs. I did not hear about any shortages of MDT while I was in Brazil. However, the medications to manage leprosy reactions and to control medication side effects were not always available. Leprosy reaction drugs such as prednisone and thalidomide are supposed to be provided free of charge as well, although there have been cases reported to MORHAN in which clinics have run out of prednisone and patients had to get these medications from a pharmacy. The shortage of prednisone at health posts may have been related to the municipalization or decentralization process of transforming the healthcare system. According to Artur Custódio de Sousa, of MORHAN, there have been problems with a lack of prednisone at some health posts since the city governments, rather than the federal government, became responsible for buying and distributing medications. Getting enough prednisone for her leprosy reactions was a problem for Sônia, forty-four. She was the only patient I spoke with who had to buy prednisone because the clinic in Niterói where she was a regular patient often ran out. She said:

> They give this medication, like I said, dapsone, these things to kill the bacilli. . . . I'm trying to do a campaign now to see if the government will help, help everyone, with prednisone. Prednisone, despite the swelling it causes, all those things—it is a way to prevent deformities. It diminishes pain. . . . And sometimes, when I have very sensitive skin, it manages to make it better. But the government doesn't have it. There's a lack; they never have it. We have to buy it.

A health official for the city of Rio de Janeiro said that prednisone should never be in short supply, although she could not speak for other clinics outside of the city limits. The health post where I spent most of my time never ran out of prednisone while I worked there.

Other medications that leprosy patients need were not always available to them free of charge, even at health posts within the city of Rio de Janeiro. Patients often had to buy the drugs for the side effects of MDT and certain experimental reaction drugs that were useful but not provided at health posts. The clinic where I conducted interviews often had extra supplies of medications they could give away to patients, but not always. Humberto, fifty, said that he bought his own medications for headaches that were probably related to MDT, and he had to buy a skin cream that "they used to give here but they don't give anymore. A different product was cheaper in the pharmacy, a cheaper cream. You have to use it on your skin—you can't stop using it."

Patrícia, twenty-two, said she usually had to buy azathioprine, a drug prescribed for her reactions, at a pharmacy in downtown Rio. She took three tablets per day, and they cost R$1.50 per tablet. One box lasted for approximately two and a half months and cost her almost R$300 (around U.S.$270 at the time). Shortly after I interviewed her, the nurse at that health post was able to find her enough extra azathioprine tablets to last her for eighteen days (about R$80 worth), as she said they were out of this medication in the pharmacy.

Marilene, twenty-four, was being treated for reaction at another clinic, but she went to the referral center where I interviewed her specifically because she heard that they had pentoxifylline available free for patients. They agreed to see her so she could get this medicine for free, because otherwise she would not have been unable to afford it. She also had to buy sedatives to help her calm down and to sleep at night. These were not that expensive, she said, but she went through the boxes of twenty pills quickly, as she took three pills a day. A health official I interviewed in June, 1999, told me that the city of Rio de Janeiro was just about to buy pentoxifylline to distribute to health posts, but they were waiting to receive a protocol for its administration from the Oswaldo Cruz Foundation, an important medical research institution in Brazil.

The lack of free medications to deal with some of the side effects of leprosy or to cope with the stress associated with having the disease or with daily life was a source of frustration for the patients who had to buy medicines on their own limited budget. Subsequent to my research in Brazil, problems related to the cost of these medications may have been alleviated for patients in some parts of Brazil. One of President Lula's signature programs is the Farmácia Popular (Popular or People's Pharmacy), intended to provide inexpensive medication for the poor (Ministério de Saúde 2005). The Oswaldo Cruz Foundation produces generic versions of many of these medications in order to make them available at a lower price. The goal was to have one thousand of these pharmacies in operation by the end of 2006, the end of Lula's first term. Several medications (including ranitidine, prednisone, and azathioprine) that patients took and sometimes had to purchase are on the list of medications available at a much discounted rate at these locations, of which there were six in the Zona Norte and Baixada Fluminense of Rio de Janeiro state as of September 2005. In addition, Rosinha Garotinho, who served as governor of the state of Rio de Janeiro from 2003 to 2007, established a program to provide many basic services, including prescriptions, for one real. Although both of these programs are arguably populist political moves (Filho 2005), they may make daily life easier for people who, like several of the patients I met, struggled to pay for medications that were not a standard part of leprosy treatment.

Patient Agency and the Medical Encounter

To reiterate a theme of this book, the patients I met and interviewed in Rio were not passive agents in their health care. They actively sought a diagnosis of their ailment and treatment of their disease and wanted to get well. The quality of the encounter with biomedicine and its representatives can affect whether or not the patient will be successful in his or her quest for health. If patients feel positive about their interactions with the public healthcare system, the treatment process tends to be easier for them, and it is more likely that they will get better more quickly. However, many patients in Brazil are repeatedly disappointed along the way as they receive misdiagnoses, have limited access to healthcare services, and experience miscommunication with doctors about medication side effects or leprosy reaction. These negative experiences can cause patients to give up on seeking treatment or to abandon treatment altogether, increasing the possibility of disability and decreasing their quality of life. I believe, however, that many patients do not give up entirely but continue to seek a resolution of their condition and a return to the way their lives were before the onset of the illness. The following chapter illustrates how different forms of stigma create problems for patients in their everyday lives.

5

Multiple Dimensions
of Leprosy Stigma

Beyond Folk Models

In Brazil as in many other parts of the world, leprosy-related stigma constitutes as much or more of a problem for affected individuals than the disease complications themselves. As leprosy is one of the more notoriously stigmatized diseases in human history, I felt it was important to include a chapter devoted to the complex nature of stigma construction and its effects on the people I met in Brazil. The predominant model of stigma in the social sciences is taken from sociologist Erving Goffman's *Stigma: Notes on the Management of Spoiled Identity*, in which he saw stigma as existing when one has "an attribute that is deeply discrediting" (1963, 3). How, though, does something come to be discrediting? Attributes that might be stigmatized are multiple, but it is difficult to identify any attributes found in human societies that are universally stigmatizing. Leprosy, for example, is not universally stigmatized, nor does leprosy stigma, where it exists, manifest in the same way cross-culturally. In some parts of Africa, very little stigma was attached to leprosy before the arrival of European missionaries (Vaughan 1991), who introduced the idea of leprosy as evidence of moral transgression. Anthropologist and physician Gilbert Lewis (1993) noted that health-care professionals in New Guinea found that stigma was not an issue in the West Sepik community where he conducted fieldwork; leprosy was rarely viewed as an illness worthy of treatment for most people who were affected. Dr. Bruce Clements of Carville commented to me in an interview (February 14, 1996):

In Micronesia, there was hardly any stigma. The children—I went
to the school to visit them, those who had leprosy. Then I went
to the homes . . . it was like it was nothing to them, no stigma at
all. They lived right with everybody else, and no one seemed to
care that it was leprosy. It didn't bother them, whereas in other
countries, of course one is India—I went there to one of the international leprosy conferences. Of course the stigma over there is
terrible. We've had some Indian patients here, immigrants who
come here who will have a lesion on their hand or foot, and they
actually ask for it to be amputated. They think that they can get
rid of the disease that way because it's such a stigma.

Anthropologists have contributed explanations that are appli-
cable to an understanding of stigma, if we can consider the relationship
between stigma and taboo. Marvin Harris (1975, 1980), who created the
explanatory paradigm of cultural materialism, explains cognitive models,
religious practices, and other culture-specific behavior in terms of the
economic advantages or disadvantages they might provide for a specific
society. He might have argued that people with certain diseases that make
them less viable members of a certain society, through various forms of
disability, may be stigmatized or constructed as dangerous. Symbolic
anthropologist Mary Douglas (1966) offered an alternative model of how
taboo and stigma are constructed. She theorized that things (e.g., animals, behaviors, diseases) that do not fit neatly into pre-existing cultural
categories are likely to be classified as symbolically unclean, polluted,
impure, or dangerous. Although leprosy is not universally constructed as
an "unclean" disease, some have argued that the characteristics of leprosy as a disease (Skinses 1964, quoted in Gussow 1989, 9), including its
long incubation period (making etiology more difficult to determine) and
the multiple deformities that can arise from untreated leprosy, have contributed to the designation of the disease as being "out of place" (Douglas
1966, 35) in many cultures' systems of illness classification.

The reasons why a particular condition, character trait, or behavior
might be stigmatized does not necessarily have to do with any inherent feature of the attribute itself; it is more about how the features
of an attribute are understood within a particular historical, cultural,

and socioeconomic context. Douglas (1991) and Foucault (1988) have argued that both the diagnosis of leprosy and the policies created to control the population of those believed to have the disease (primarily the poor) in medieval Europe were intimately connected to the social, political, and religious hierarchies that existed during that time. Zachary Gussow (1989) has emphasized the role of European colonialism in the reemergence of leprosy stigma and a new leprosarium era toward the end of the nineteenth century. According to Gussow (1989, 19–20), "The late nineteenth-century Western opinion that leprosy was highly contagious . . . was not formed through extended observation and careful studies of the behavior of the disease. Rather, it was formed by the general attitudes held in Western nations about the character and the symbolic attributes supposedly possessed by the colonial populations in which the disease was presumed to be inherent."

Inequalities or political tension within a society might be a major factor in how and whether stigma will be constructed. Richard Parker and Peter Aggleton (2003), an anthropologist and sociologist, respectively, have pointed out that stigma cannot be divorced from the structural inequalities that exist in the society in which it is felt or enacted. In the contemporary context, leprosy stigma and the perception of this stigma continue to be influenced by a web of interconnected factors that affect the lives of people with this disease. In 2004, at an international workshop on health-related stigma, sponsored by Holland's Royal Tropical Institute and held in Soesterberg, Holland, I was in a group given the task of constructing "models" for understanding stigma. We discussed at length the numerous factors that cannot be ignored when looking at stigma, where it comes from, and how to combat it. We made lists of dozens of factors (including class structure, gender roles, religious beliefs, patterns of daily life in the culture in question, local perceptions about the body and health, how treatment is administered, side effects of treatment, and many more) that have each had an impact on stigma individually and that constantly interact with each other to shape ideas about disease and health. Although the model we came up with provided a potential framework for looking at stigma in any context, each stigmatizing condition must be viewed individually in its particular geographical and cultural setting.

Leprosy Stigma in Brazil

Fear of leprosy in the general population in Brazil was pronounced in the early twentieth century, but once the leprosarium era began, this fear seemed to have more to do with mandatory isolation policies than with the potential effects of the disease. Within the leprosaria in Brazil and elsewhere, the idea of leprosy as a contaminating and unclean disease was promoted by the physical confinement of the facilities and by the treatment of patients, modeled, in part, on the system of isolation of leprosy patients in the United States. In a leprosarium in southern Brazil, for example, the patients' area of residence was referred to as the *área suja* (dirty area) and the staff area as the *área limpo* (clean area). This leprosarium also issued its own inter-facility coins for patients to use, which both reflected and perpetuated fears that leprosy was inordinately contagious (Fontoura, Barcelos, and Borges 2003).

Today, leprosy is treated on an outpatient basis and, as mentioned in previous chapters, is most common among people of the lower socioeconomic classes in Brazil (in both urban and rural areas). This population is one that is already stigmatized as "marginal" or "dangerous." Nancy Scheper-Hughes (1992) notes that there is a continued depiction of both favela residents and street children in Brazil as "dirty" from the perspective of the middle and upper classes. The fact that leprosy and other contagious diseases are more common among Brazil's lower socioeconomic classes reinforces the idea held by people of the upper classes that these segments of the population are sources of contamination and marks leprosy as a disease of the poor.

The current picture of stigma surrounding leprosy in Brazil is complex. There are elements of the medieval and biblical understandings of leprosy, although European models of disease and the body in general were also mixed with West African, and to some extent, indigenous South American models. The existence of and knowledge about leprosaria within the country (as mentioned in chapter 2, thirty-three former leprosaria with former patient residents still exist in Brazil today) contributes to beliefs about contagion and the necessity of isolation. Popular media and popular religion also provide images and ideas about leprosy in Brazil. According to one of the physicians I interviewed, people in Brazil are "afraid of the disabilities that hanseníase could bring—not just physical but moral [disability]. Because if you say you have hanseníase, someone else might imagine that you are impure and unclean, which elicits loathing and disgust."

The campaign to change the name from *lepra* to *hanseníase* has been a successful one in Brazil, though, as mentioned earlier, this has not necessarily reduced stigma among those who know little about either disease. In beginning my fieldwork in Brazil, I did not encounter significant fear associated with either lepra or hanseníase among middle-class Brazilians I spoke with; for the most part, people were surprised that it was still such a problem in Brazil. However, fear cannot necessarily be measured by reaction to a discussion of a disease. My first personal encounter with a strong fear-based reaction to contact with leprosy patients occurred when a television producer from the United States came to film a Discovery Channel documentary (Ward 1999) about leprosy. She hired a Brazil-based camera crew. The chief cameraman (who was German) initially quit the assignment because his Brazilian wife, a doctor, was afraid the disease was highly contagious, and she was afraid of contamination of their young child. After learning a little more about the disease, he changed his mind and continued with the project.

In Portuguese, the word that is more frequently used by the general public to talk about stigma is *preconceito*, or preconception—preconceived ideas about what leprosy is or about a person who appears to be ill. Leprosy patients may encounter stigmatization from many different sources, including friends, relatives, employers, neighbors, and people they meet on the street. In my interviews with patients, one of my original questions was, "Do you tell your family, friends, employer about your disease?" Artur Custódio de Sousa, of MORHAN, reviewed my interview questions before I began research, and he suggested that I break this question down into three separate ones. Patients talk about their illness with people among whom they have primary relationships, particularly family and close friends, but they are less likely to want to share this information with mere acquaintances or colleagues at work.

Often when I asked patients about stigma in their community, they said they had not experienced it, but "*poucos sabem*" (few know)

about their disease. Outpatient treatment, in contrast to the mandatory isolation of the past, facilitates concealment of leprosy. Also,
most patients I saw have no obvious signs of disease. They might have
a few discolored patches of skin under their clothes. They may have
problems with their hands or feet, but in many cases, there is nothing
that would signal "leprosy" to the general public. In the case of visible
lesions or spots on the skin, many patients, when asked by strangers
or acquaintances about what was wrong with them, responded that it
was "from the beach," that it was an allergy, or that it was a fungus,
and people tended to be satisfied with that answer. Doctors and social
workers often recommend that patients be cautious about revealing
their disease to others.

Nine patients I interviewed said they did not tell anyone beyond
family members about their disease. Others told friends but usually
only the close friends they felt they could trust. Three patients said that
they told non-family members about their disease only if they noticed
possible symptoms of leprosy in the person and wanted to encourage
them to seek a diagnosis. The reason patients do not reveal their illness is primarily that they do not want people to be suspicious of them,
fear them, or stigmatize them. For example, Denise, twenty-seven, said
she decided not tell to anyone outside of the family about her disease
because "where I live . . . the people just think nonsense." They would
associate leprosy with many things that have "nothing to do with" the
disease. She believed that patients who choose to reveal their diagnosis
risk various forms of stigma. Because of illness concealment, only a few
patients experienced stigma from the outside world, but several developed self-stigmatizing behaviors or feelings that affected their social
life and mental well-being. Below, I have organized patient accounts of
perceived stigma in terms of the types of relationships and settings in
which the stigma was experienced.

Stigma on the Job

Although it is not legal in Brazil to fire someone for having leprosy,
patients still run the risk of losing their job if they reveal their disease
to their employer. Only four patients I talked to, though, claimed to

have experienced stigma in the workplace. Two of these patients were fired because of their illness. These numbers might be low because many patients simply did not tell anyone at work they had leprosy. Others were fortunate enough to have enlightened employers. Although most people said they did not tell colleagues at work about their disease, patients were often obliged to reveal to their employer that they were being treated for leprosy, particularly if they had to miss work because of illness or because of clinic appointments. Several patients told me that their *firmas* (company or corporation) had a doctor, and these company doctors would be the ones to receive the information about their illness. In some cases, these doctors would be understanding and helpful. Afonso, fifty-one, who was working as a welder, had a good experience:

C.W.: Did you ever have a problem coming here [missing work]?

AFONSO: No, and I even spoke with my department—[with] the people there—and told them I'm in treatment. I think they know that I have this disease because the doctor there at my work has a [position] at a health post. So she must know about this problem.

Gerson, twenty-three, who built buses for a living, experienced more of a problem at work:

In the first company [where I was working] when I had the disease, they avoided me. Then they said, "Send him away." [That was] the first company. Then I stayed quiet. . . . The company doctor sent me away, because of this, because of the stigma. You know that this person is sick, everyone's asking, then no one wants to work with me. This is why they sent me away. They won't let me work because of people's stigma.

It was clear from Gerson's comment that his employers were blaming his fellow employees' fear on their decision to let him go, rather than, for example, providing a brief educational session for employees about the fact that a person does not transmit leprosy once he or she has begun treatment. In another example, a woman who worked as a coffee server at a museum in Niterói, a satellite city across the bay from Rio, contacted MORHAN because she had been suspended from work.

MORHAN was able to give a talk to the museum staff to educate them about leprosy and allay their fears.

Laura, a patient in her mid-forties, was working at, ironically, an institution for medical research. Despite the availability of medical information at her place of employment, as well as the existence of an outpatient treatment center for leprosy on the grounds of the facility, her manager was very fearful of leprosy. She told her, "Look, if it were up to me, you would be leaving today because this disease is contagious. I have a son and a husband, and I don't want you to stay." Laura was able to recruit a social worker from the same institution to help her keep her job.

Patients who do not have contact with a helpful clinic staff or NGO may have very little recourse if they lose their job because of leprosy. Patients working in the informal economy are particularly vulnerable. Based on my interviews with patients and on my analysis of phone calls to MORHAN's informational phone line, Telehansen, it seems that patients who work in private homes for middle- and upper-class families in Rio are in a particularly precarious position with regard to their jobs if they reveal to their employer that they have leprosy. Maids, nannies, gardeners, cooks, and other domestic servants work in close contact with the family that employs them as well as with the personal items used by the family. Several calls to Telehansen revealed a preoccupation about contagion among employers of domestic workers. One woman called to say she had a person working in her house who had symptoms that were the same as those she had seen on a flier (distributed by MORHAN) and wondered if it could be leprosy; this could be interpreted either as concern for an employees' health or a preoccupation with the health and safety of the caller (and perhaps her family). Another caller stated that the caretaker of his garden had leprosy and asked if it was possible to contract the disease through the garden. A MORHAN volunteer told me about another Telehansen call: "A woman called last week [and said]: 'I have a bricklayer/mason [pedreiro] who has this disease. It's just that every time he leaves I have to rub alcohol on the masonry, rub alcohol on the floor where he stepped.' So, we have to explain to her what the disease is like . . . that it doesn't present a danger in that way." In some cases, employers of domestic workers do not bother to learn more about the disease. They simply fire their employees outright. Regina, thirty-four, was a domestic worker until she was diagnosed with leprosy, after which she was immediately fired: "I worked there six years, but then I became a problem for her . . . she had children and didn't even want to talk to me. She sent me away because of the children."

Stigma against leprosy in the workplace can create much anxiety in patients' daily lives. It threatens their job security and their ability to provide for their families. If colleagues hold stigmatizing attitudes, patients experience isolation and ostracism at work. Patients with no obvious symptoms thus often do not reveal their illness to employers and colleagues in order to avoid stigma.

Friends, Neighbors, Acquaintances

Patients who experienced stigma in public or in their own community usually had visible signs of the disease or problems with leprosy reaction that resulted in lesions. Sometimes the medications also caused changes in appearance. Eight patients, about a fifth of those patients I interviewed, had experienced stigma from friends, neighbors, and/or people in their community. From the patients' perspectives, stigma consisted of others remarking on or reacting to lesions or other visible physical abnormalities. It is important to point out that patients felt stigmatized not because they had leprosy specifically, but because the physical signs of leprosy drew unwanted attention and questions. This may be related to a fear in the general population of contagious disease in general. Although questions about skin changes may be viewed as stigmatizing by patients, it may be simple curiosity or concern on the part of others.

Gerson, twenty-three, was made to feel uncomfortable by people's comments about his appearance. He said he had to stop going outside without wearing his shirt because people would ask him about his skin. He discovered that trying to explain his disease could also be stigmatizing:

GERSON: My shoulders were all spotted, and people would ask me what it was.
C.W.: What do you tell people?

GERSON: I said it was hanseníase but no one understood what that was. You couldn't say lepra because they avoid you. People are very ignorant. They don't know the disease and the studies [about it]. They don't know, and they would avoid me, stay away from me.

Daniela, nineteen, who was undergoing a severe reaction at the time of interview, with red pockmarks up and down her arms and legs, said that her family supported her but "all of my friends distanced themselves from me." They were afraid that it was contagious, she said. She also said that she has not been able to get a job because of her appearance, so she helps out at home. Stigma based on her changed appearance was severe enough to prevent her from socializing and achieving independence.

Fernando, twenty, did not reveal to his friends that he had leprosy, but his aunt did, which prompted a large fight between his aunt and his mother and grandmother, who thought it was a bad idea to reveal the diagnosis. I asked him if his friends still accepted him:

FERNANDO: They did. They were sad.
C.W.: No one was afraid?
FERNANDO: They thought I was going to die. Then they started to treat me differently . . . like I was going to die.

In Fernando's case, it appears that his friends were concerned not because they held stigmatizing attitudes about leprosy; they treated him differently because they thought he had a life-threatening disease (which leprosy is not)—this can feel stigmatizing to the recipient of such treatment, but it is not specifically leprosy-related stigma.

With acquaintances, just as with colleagues and employers, most patients whose symptoms are not very obvious do not reveal anything at all about their disease and thus generally do not experience stigma. *Não costumo falar* (I don't usually talk about it) was the most common way patients expressed their chosen silence about the disease. Humberto, fifty, says he approaches people who he thinks might have the disease, but he does not usually tell people otherwise: "Because if you talk to just anyone who doesn't understand, who you don't know, certainly they'll have a different reaction. They'll want to get away from you, surely." Certainly, beyond very close friends and family, many patients felt that revealing the disease would be foolish and that there is no point in telling acquaintances when they were already in treatment and their disease was no longer contagious.

Stigma among Family Members

Family ties in Brazil are usually very important. Based on my observations, family members take care of each other and form very close-knit ties. Anthropologist Charles Wagley wrote, "The persistence of the widely extended *parentela* [kinship group] in Brazil must be considered as the reflection of deep-seated Luso-Brazilian values. The patriarchal family system of the plantation era may have disappeared, yet the strong bonds of kinship have been re-formed in terms of contemporary conditions of life" (1995, 149). Contrary to stereotypes of marginality in Brazil, people in lower socioeconomic classes also maintain strong social ties. Cynthia Sarti worked in low-income neighborhoods of São Paulo and studied morality and family life. She has written that "in hard times the poor rely on reciprocal family relations to help each other—as in times of sickness or when a newly arrived relative is becoming established in the city. In fact, there is [a] sense of obligation, but rooted in the principle of reciprocity and complementarity that structures family life and within which affection is developed" (Sarti 1995, 120).

Among my sample, leprosy did not seem to be a motivation for families to abandon a family member with the disease. Most patients I spoke with were strongly supported by their families. Other studies of leprosy patients in Rio de Janeiro also have shown that families generally are supportive of patients. Rita Pereira, a social worker, did a small study of fourteen women affected by leprosy in Rio de Janeiro and found that the women who were married neither separated themselves from their families nor suffered stigmatization from their husbands or children (Pereira 1996). In Lenita Claro's study of leprosy patients in Rio, most patients who decided not to reveal their diagnosis to everyone they knew still trusted family members with this information (1995, 94). A few patients I interviewed experienced some initial stigma from their spouses, usually husbands, but eventually they ceased having fears or doubts after talking to physicians or social workers. Alícia, thirty-nine, told me: "My husband was ashamed. . . . We have two kids, and he was afraid for them. . . . He was a little [nervous] about it. Always afraid. But I brought him here [to the clinic] and now it's fine."

In personal communication with Pereira, she told me that she believes that families do not abandon other family members because of leprosy unless there were strained relationships prior to the diagnosis. One example she gave of this was a man who came to a self-help group at a health post where she was working. He had separated himself completely from his family, and his family kept their distance from him. When he found out he had leprosy, he began to live separately from them, but in an adjacent house, and he kept his utensils and other items separate. However, when a social worker offered to visit his family, he said that he never got along with them to begin with, and he was not interested in having them learn more about his disease.

Six of the patients I interviewed mentioned some form of stigmatization from relatives. For two patients, the relatives were somewhat distant relations, as with Ximena, age fifty, who said she felt stigmatized by her husband's family. Three of these six had a husband or wife who was afraid of the disease at first but later changed their attitude. Only one patient, Manoel, thirty, was abandoned by some family members and friends; his case is discussed in more depth in the next chapter, but it is important to note that none of the people who abandoned him did so specifically because of leprosy. He attributed the abandonment more to the loss of earning potential due to leprosy-related disability than to others' fear of leprosy (particularly since no one recognized his disease as leprosy).

Though healthcare workers and volunteers I spoke with were aware of cases of abandonment or stigmatization of patients by close relatives in Brazil because of leprosy, the patients I talked to generally received a great deal of support from children, wives, husbands, and parents. In part, this is related to the fact that patients are treated on an outpatient basis and are not isolated from their relatives. In the past, long-term isolation and institutionalization led to alienation from family members. The incurability of the disease before the development of sulfone drugs was also a factor in family stigmatization of patients.

Today, patients are able to demonstrate to their relatives that leprosy is curable, and treatment is much simpler because patients come into the clinic once a month and are able to bring their medications home, so patients are able to maintain family ties.

Self-Stigmatization

Lenita Claro, in her study of leprosy patients in Rio de Janeiro, wrote that contrary to her research team's original hypothesis that many patients with leprosy had experienced stigma related to their disease, stigma was not a problem for the majority of patients who were interviewed: "On the contrary, self-stigmatization was revealed as a central issue for some of the patients" (1995, 86). Although patients do make observations about people's behaviors and attitudes about leprosy and are correct to think that a stigma against lepra exists, they deprive others of the opportunity to show acceptance by stigmatizing and isolating themselves, though at the same time, reasonably, protecting themselves from the possible stigmatizing attitudes that some people might hold. The patients I interviewed who were not afraid to talk about their disease and who actively sought support among their family and friends did not experience stigma. Although most patients were able to conceal their illness from others if they chose to do so, many self-stigmatized. For some, self-stigmatization was related to an initial fear that leprosy was contagious. For others, it was related instead to a loss of self-esteem due to the physical effects of the disease or the medications. Thus, some patients also chose to go beyond keeping their illness a secret and actively distanced themselves from friends and stopped leaving the house.

Patrícia, twenty-two, isolated herself from much of the world when she found out she had leprosy. She and her boyfriend had broken up around the same time she found out she had the disease. But her self-stigmatization was related, in part, to the effects of the steroids she was taking for leprosy reaction:

> I had done everything with him—shopping, movies, going out—everything with him. Then I started leaving my friends behind. I lost friendships. His friends were my friends. Then

when I found out I had hanseníase, I started to gain weight. And this was combined with the friendships I didn't have. The fat complex, right? So I just had my mother, my father, my colleagues from work—who were really [just] colleagues, not really the same as friends.

Her weight gain increased with high doses of prednisone, and she stopped going out. She also changed her job to one that was more compatible with her clinic visits, so now she has even fewer friends. She anticipated, however, that had she revealed her diagnosis to others, she would have experienced stigma:

I just hid, as much as I could. But I think that if I talked about it, there would be stigma. There would be. And people don't know how you get it, but many don't want to know. They don't want to run the risk of getting it. I also closed myself off a lot. My dad will say, "Let's go eat with a friend," or whatever [but I don't go], I was always a homebody, so this helps me even more [to avoid stigma]."

In addition to the emotional and economic consequences of stigma, self-stigmatization can also affect patient adherence to medication as well as the decision to seek treatment in the first place. In India, for example, where leprosy is both more common than in Brazil and more highly stigmatized (and perhaps more likely to be recognized in its early stages by patients themselves), delay in treatment-seeking behavior because of anticipated stigma has been documented. Ron Barrett (2005) has described how fear of stigmatization and concealment of symptoms prevents patients from getting treatment; as a result, many patients develop severe deformities and disabilities that could have been prevented with MDT. In Brazil, examples of leprosy stigma (in other words, stigma that is directly related to "lepra" or "hanseníase") were less common in my own research; such cases tend to occur in Brazil where there is an awareness of or direct contact with (on the part of patients or others with whom the patient interacts) communities that once served as leprosaria, where former patients and their families often continue to live today.

The American Leprosy Missions Brazil (2005) Web site contains several brief life histories of patients. One, "J.R.S.," thirty-four years old, was diagnosed with leprosy when he was a teenager, but he neither sought treatment nor revealed his diagnosis to anyone. His father had leprosy, and he lived with his father on the grounds of a former leprosarium. Having perceived that his father was stigmatized for his illness, he felt that the treatment (and thus, the revelation of his illness to the world) would result in his being stigmatized by friends. The association of leprosy with isolation may still be salient in the minds of the children and grandchildren of people who were forcibly institutionalized after being diagnosed with leprosy.

In another example, Suzana Duran, a psychologist at a facility that formerly operated as a leprosarium and that is currently an outpatient treatment center for leprosy and other diseases, gave me her report (Duran 1995) on the case of SER (a pseudonym that means, in Portuguese, "to be," and that is also the acronym "Social and Economic Rehabilitation"), a boy whose mother had been diagnosed with leprosy at this facility. The woman met a resident there who encouraged her to cut off her ties with the outside world, move onto the grounds of the facility (where, at the time, housing and new construction were relatively unregulated by the administration), and accept her status as a "leper." She stopped taking MDT, convinced that leprosy was incurable. Her son, SER, was also diagnosed with leprosy and experienced stigma from classmates and parents of classmates at the public school he attended because there were visible manifestations of his illness and it was known that he lived on the grounds of the treatment facility. Ultimately, an intervention at the school and with the mother was designed, but it is clear that the presence of this facility and the legacy of the leprosarium era result in a perpetuation of stigma and in self-stigmatization and even, in the case of SER's mother, self-institutionalization for a curable disease.

Addressing Stigma

One might argue that the simplest way to ensure that stigma associated with leprosy does not continue to be a problem would be to ensure that leprosy itself be eradicated. However, in Brazil, even if no new cases of leprosy were detected, there would still be hundreds of thousands of individuals who have been "cured" of leprosy but who may continue to suffer stigma resulting from disabilities associated with the disease or from preconceptions in the general populace about leprosy. Thus, stigma is something that needs to be a part of leprosy-control programs. The renaming of the disease to hanseníase has had some effect in reducing stigma (particularly self-stigmatization), as has the emphasis on the curability of hanseníase. Perhaps improvements in the treatment regimen designed to reduce medication side effects that are visible might diminish perceived stigma for patients. Iatrogenic stigma, or that which is generated through the discourse, procedures, and loci of the medical encounter, is also an important area of focus in leprosy treatment (White 2007). Education is also an important component, but education campaigns must be carefully constructed. Biomedical information about stigma might in some cases increase fear associated with leprosy (Staples 2004); for example, the biomedical model in which leprosy is an infectious-contagious disease that can be transmitted from person to person through breathing might generate more fear and stigma than the Brazilian folk model in which leprosy comes from dogs. Campaigns that emphasize the curability of hanseníase may be positive in reducing stigma and encouraging people to seek treatment. I will discuss public education and "social marketing" campaigns in chapter 7.

An example of how stigmatizing attitudes with multiple consequences can be overcome in a relatively short period of time was described to me by a psychologist and MORHAN volunteer I interviewed. A woman had overheard people talking on a bus about a leprosy patient in her community. The woman found out where this person lived and went there herself. She found that there was an elderly woman locked in her room. Her family gave her food through a hole in the door, and she had a bathroom in the room. The elderly woman was in treatment for leprosy, but "she only left her room to go to the health post, and the family was afraid to ask about hanseníase. They just picked up her medicines and returned home." The woman who had looked into this situation called MORHAN, and they visited the house. The psychologist told me the following story:

I talked with her daughter and one of the grown grandchildren and we started to talk about what hanseníase was. And I brought some photos for her to be able to identify [the disease] by seeing the photos. That was when she told me that her mother had hanseníase, but she thought it was difficult to cure since she had many reactions. Then I asked her to call the woman, and she went there and opened the door and the woman came out. And other children were coming in and even a neighbor came in, and I started talking about hanseníase. It was then that the daughter asked her mother to sit next to her. I think this was the most important part because they were able to break that stigma, that fear they had of her. And then the granddaughter allowed her baby to sit near its great-grandmother. She did not even know about the existence of some of these other grandchildren and great-grandchildren.

In a matter of minutes, in this case, the stigmatizing behaviors of this family were dismantled. This story illustrates the importance of disseminating information about leprosy when patients come in for treatment.

6

The Contemporary
Experience of Leprosy

Five Narratives

The most interesting, most rewarding, and sometimes most difficult part of my research occurred in the process of listening to patients' stories about their experiences with leprosy. The interview questions I put together were meant to elicit illness narratives from patients and were organized chronologically, from first appearance of symptoms, to diagnosis, to treatment, to, in some cases, cure and post-cure. I found that the people I spoke with who were affected by leprosy, some of whom I had met only minutes before the interview, were incredibly open and generous in sharing very personal and painful memories with a virtual stranger. Many had clearly reflected on their illness but perhaps never discussed it fully. A few cried as they recounted their experiences, not only with the disease and its complications, but also with other aspects of their lives that had been difficult.

In this chapter, I present the illness narratives of five of the people I interviewed, whose lives were affected by having leprosy in Rio de Janeiro, Brazil. Their stories are assembled from the tape-recorded interviews I conducted with them (using the questions in Appendix A as a starting point) and, in some cases, from additional informal conversations and my observations of their experiences with treatment. As mentioned above, my interviewees were at different stages of treatment for leprosy, but because the outpatient treatment center where I spent most of my time was a referral center for complicated cases, many people had completed MDT but continued to suffer from problems associated with leprosy reaction. I have attempted to include the stories of patients who, together, represent a range of experiences with leprosy and leprosy treatment in Brazil. The economic struggles and the conditions of daily life described in these narratives are representative of those of all the patients I interviewed.

At the aforementioned stigma workshop I attended in the Netherlands in 2004, some of the participants pointed out that focusing on patients' positive experiences and "success stories," rather than always looking at the examples of stigma, discrimination, and suffering, might be a useful exercise. Medical anthropologist Susan McCombie, my colleague at Georgia State University, has encouraged me to highlight what has worked for patients and to consider how their experiences can be replicated. I have tried to incorporate these suggestions into my approach to examining patients' experiences with leprosy in general. While it is important to acknowledge and describe the problems people encounter and the suffering they endure, it is equally important to look at the cases in which people have successfully negotiated the treatment program with minimal difficulty or impact on their lives. We can then try to look at what is unique about their cases to see if there are lessons we can learn that could be used to improve the experience of leprosy for others in Brazil and elsewhere. In some senses, all of the cases described below are "success stories" because they represent the narratives of individuals who have been able to get treatment for leprosy and have found various effective coping mechanisms for living with the consequences of the disease. However, some encountered much greater hardship and suffering along the way than others. I chose to include these narratives not simply because they are interesting vignettes that provide some insight into daily life for low-income individuals in Brazilian society but also because, in their stories, there are indications of some of the problems patients affected by leprosy in Brazil experienced during the time I conducted my research. From an applied anthropological perspective, the collection and analysis of patient narratives, coupled with observations in the health post, can be used to inform policy decisions regarding treatment for infectious diseases with complicated treatment programs.

Sônia

I first met Sônia in 1995, on my preliminary research trip to Rio, in the offices of MORHAN. She had just completed two years of treatment with MDT for multibacillary leprosy and was thus "cured" from a biomedical standpoint, and she had begun volunteering for MORHAN. However, she was still having problems with leprosy reaction, which she expressed concern about at the time. She had no visible disabilities, but I noted in my fieldnotes then that she seemed to have some skin pigmentation problems (from the drug clofazimine). I met her again in 1998 at an outpatient treatment center; after speaking with her for a few minutes, we realized we had met before, and she agreed to do an interview with me. She was still volunteering for MORHAN, so we set up the interview at the offices of this NGO rather than at the clinic. When I conducted my interview with her, she was forty-four years old, divorced, with two grown children, both married. She was having severe reactions (fever, pain, new lesions, and nerve damage) and had become quite frustrated that she was not yet well.

Sônia first started having leprosy-related problems at age thirty-six: "I had a lot of pain. I couldn't take a step. It hurt a lot, I wasn't walking. I swelled up. My feet, hands, and nose were swelling. There was a lot of congestion in my nose that made breathing difficult." She was misdiagnosed as having arthritis and was put on a medication regime for that. Because of the nerve involvement and subsequent problems with hands and feet, arthritis is a common misdiagnosis given to people with leprosy. Then, she said, the doctors thought she had syphilis. While taking the syphilis treatment (Bencetazil, she said, which is a brand name for benzathine penicillin), lesions began to appear on her back. It was only once these characteristic lesions appeared that a private doctor suspected she might have leprosy and sent her to a dermatologist, where, she said, "The doctor said I had hansen":

> For me it was a real impact when I found out. My diagnosis was, "You have hanseníase." I didn't know [what that was]. She didn't even tell me that hanseníase is lepra. I thought I had cancer . . . I was terrified.

As mentioned in chapter 3, the word *hanseníase*, a Brazilianized version of a foreign name, was not easily understood by patients hearing it for the first time. *Hansen* and *cancer* also sound quite similar. Sônia said that her physician suggested she hide the fact that she had hanseníase from others:

> She told me I shouldn't tell anyone . . . that I shouldn't talk to people that don't have any knowledge because it's a contagious disease. . . . So because I'm very contrary, I did the opposite of what she said. I told my friends. I arrived home very upset, thinking it was cancer. And to my friend, a very close friend, I said, "Look, I have this disease." And she started to cheer me up, saying that it had a cure.

Though Sônia was willing to talk about her illness openly, she did not accept her diagnosis of leprosy initially, in part because she had been misdiagnosed in the past. Also, after she began treatment for leprosy, she told me that her doctors said they were finding more bacilli than before in her skin scrapings and biopsies, so she suspected something else was wrong with her. The large number of bacilli in her body led her to have numerous episodes of leprosy reaction. So despite the treatment, she was feeling worse than ever: "Even three months into the treatment, I didn't want to accept that I had hanseníase."

Both from her experiences in outpatient treatment for leprosy and from her work as a volunteer for MORHAN, Sônia had become familiar with the biomedical model of leprosy. She could name the MDT medications and knew that she had a form of multibacillary leprosy (she used the term "hanseníase *virchowiana*," known in English as lepromatous leprosy), for which she took twenty-four doses of MDT. She mentioned "lowered immunity" as a root cause of her getting leprosy and thought that malnutrition, or undernutrition, may have made her more susceptible to the disease, particularly during a time when she was married and her husband "had a very hard head. He wouldn't let me work, and he couldn't earn enough. So, I think that all this compromises [one's immune system]." However, some of her speculations on the etiological agent of leprosy contrasted with the medical model. She thought she might have caught the disease from the open ditch or sewer (*valão*) near her house in her favela neighborhood: "I lived breathing that air from the sewer every day." She also speculated that she could have been exposed to it on the job. Before getting married, she had worked as a cleaning woman, washing floors and cleaning bathrooms in hotels and department stores, and she had to breathe in a lot of dust and dirt. "In other words," she told me, as she concluded her speculations on etiology, "I've had plenty of opportunities to catch hanseníase. . . . What do you think?" she asked me, at which point I discussed the biomedical model with her. She also considered the possibility that God may have given her this disease not as a punishment, but for the purpose of changing her life for the better.

Medication side effects were a major problem for Sônia. She expressed her problems with the change in skin tone that comes from the drug clofazimine, which she took for two years. She described herself as "very vain. . . . Every woman is, right? So you live in a neighborhood, you feel scandalized by people's gaze, you know?" She had once been pale, she said, but she noted that her skin turned several shades darker with clofazimine. She said that it was not apparent to strangers, but her acquaintances noticed and commented that something strange was happening to her. People in her neighborhood began to ask her questions: "Why are you black like that? What is that?" As Sônia said, "With my dark face, it was a scandal, but only for those who knew me. For those who didn't know me, it wasn't a scandal because my appearance was healthy."

Sônia noticed that when she was upset or anxious, her physical problems were made worse: "I have many emotional problems, a lot of frustrations—so it could be that this affects the pains in my nerves. I think so, you know? . . . Because when I have any type of frustration, I feel more pains." A social worker I worked with in Brazil conducted a small study to try to demonstrate that there was a correlation between personal stress and incidence of leprosy reaction in women (Pereira 1996). People who suffer from leprosy reaction are believed to have depressed immune function; multiple studies have demonstrated that chronic emotional stress for people whose immune systems are already compromised in some way can have a negative effect on disease outcome (Segerstrom and Miller 2004).

Sônia, whose economic situation was precarious before her diagnosis, had many different sources of stress in her life, and her illness exacerbated many of her problems. While she suffered from leprosy reactions, it was impossible for her to work. She became completely dependent on others for food and for medicines that were not provided free of charge. She said it was very difficult: "I'm a humble person, but . . . I have my limits," she said. Before getting sick, she was poor, but, she said:

> I had money to buy my clothes, to feed my children . . . I never
> imagined I would be living on one minimum salary [equivalent
> to about seventy dollars U.S. per month at the time of the inter-
> view]. . . . I used to think, how do people live on a minimum
> salary? And now I do. Understand? I've lived on less. I worked
> two times a week in a house before I found out I had hanseníase,
> earning half a minimum salary. Half. It was the worst time in my
> life. I had bread in the morning and I had to arrange something
> in the afternoon. . . . But even earning minimum wage, I wind
> up depending on other people for medicines, even today, on the
> church. I get depressed. They say, "You shouldn't be this way.
> We're here to help you." Also, my house is terrible. The roof—it's
> an old apartment. It rains in. . . . I have to ask my sister for
> money. I get depressed, depending on others.

After she began having leprosy-related problems but before she received her diagnosis, Sônia converted to evangelical Protestantism. She told me about her spiritual transformation: "Before I was a Catholic, like many say they are. Catholic-Spiritist. . . . You say you're Catholic but you go to a Spiritist center. So, I was an open Catholic. But when Jesus entered my life, everything changed." She was working in a house as a maid of a woman who was a friend of her family's. The woman let Sônia stay there after Sônia separated from her husband. This woman was evangelical:

> I had a lot of pain, and I was taking all these medicines. She
> invited me to go to her church. . . . It was my first meeting/
> encounter [*encontro*] with Jesus. . . . At first I didn't want it

because I thought it was tiresome. . . . I drank, I smoked, all these things that I thought I had to have in my life. . . . But I accepted it. When I accepted it was when I discovered what [disease] I had.

Her church proved to be a source of much support, both emotional and financial, during her illness. At one health post, Sônia was given the drug pentoxifylline, and she was very pleased with the effectiveness of this drug for her reactions. Pentoxifylline, however, is not universally distributed to health posts where leprosy is treated in Brazil because it is quite costly. "Trental [a brand name for pentoxifylline] costs twenty-one or twenty-two reals per box. But it only has twenty pills. I have to buy five boxes a month. I earn minimum wage—120 or 130 reals. How can I buy this medicine?" She was also taking a medication called Dilex, presumably for asthma, which cost her about thirty reals per week. In order to keep buying her medications, Sônia sought help in her church and through an evangelical radio station:

I wrote them a letter. . . . They read my letter on the air, and then people sent me medicines. They sent medicines to me, and I had enough medicines for two months. Then afterwards, I couldn't afford them again. I asked again on the radio. The church helps me with these medicines too. It's been a year that my church buys these medicines for me.

People from her church also helped her by providing her with food, because, as she said, "In my house it's not possible to buy food" on her government pension, equivalent to one minimum wage. The support she has received from her church also secured her faith:

Look, my encounter with Jesus has been marvelous because the church—my church has helped me. How? It buys my medicines, it helps me with food . . . in everything it's helped me. . . . My church has helped me spiritually, the strength that all the brothers and sisters give to feel better, to feel that you're going to get better, that [the problems are] not going to continue.

She contrasted the optimism about her health expressed by fellow church members to the ways that doctors have talked about her case.

Doctors often told her they did not know what to do next for her. They would tell her how "complicated" her case was. "They say I'm a pain [*uma chatinha*]." Her own and her doctors' frustrations with her repeated bouts with leprosy reaction prompted her to briefly abandon her treatment program. Fellow church members also suggested to her that this might be a good option. She had observed that when her neighbors prayed over her open sores, they would close up the following day. So she decided to stop taking her medicines altogether:

> One day, I said to God, "God, I can't take anymore. I just take medicines and never stop. I take a lot of medicines. A lot of things. So . . . I'm not going to take any more . . ." I stopped taking the medicines, and I got very sick. I was in horrible shape. The pains were worse than ever. I stayed in bed. I spoke in shouts . . . and the wounds—I had sores all over. . . . That's not what I wanted. I went back to taking the medicines.

C.W.: How long did you stop? A week?

SÔNIA: No, I stopped for a day. You can't stop. . . . Because I was taking sixty milligrams [of prednisone per day]—you stop, you risk your life.

Because prednisone requires a slow tapering off of the dosage in ten-milligram increments per week, it is very dangerous, from a biomedical standpoint, to stop taking this medicine all of a sudden, which Sônia discovered from her experience. "There are people who believe that Jesus cures you, and they stop taking their medications. In my life, it hasn't worked that way." Though she believes that God and Jesus are ultimately responsible for restoring health, she now believes that they work by providing you with the medical options to get better.

Although her case was a difficult one, Sônia said that overall she had had very positive experiences with the physicians who had treated her for leprosy and leprosy reaction. She had one doctor who made house calls when she was too poor to buy medications and too sick from leprosy reaction to come into the clinic:

> He looked for me at home and treated me at home, in Niterói. So I thank [this doctor], you know, because he said I was deserving. I said, "No, I don't deserve anything." He has real love. He came

to my house, there on the hill [*morro*, which is often synonymous
with favela], you know. He even bought skin cream for me. . . .
He gave me medication for my blood pressure, because I had
been taking prednisone for a long time, and it gives you poor
circulation.

Sônia was struggling on many levels—emotional, financial, and
physical—when I interviewed her. Her problems with leprosy reaction
were ongoing, despite having completed MDT many years ago, and leprosy reaction continued to affect her ability to work. She was dependent
on others for her housing, food, and medicines. However, she was also
very proactive in her approach to her illness. She did not keep her illness a secret, and as a vocal person, she managed to create support networks for herself and circumvent leprosy-related stigma. She had told
her friends, family, and people in her church that she had leprosy: "All
my friends support me, and in my neighborhood, everyone knows I had
hanseníase. That's why I told you you can publish my name—because
I insist that people see. I don't have any fear." I chose to use a pseudonym for her, though I have disguised little else about her identity.
She had given lectures to public school students about leprosy and had
appeared in interviews arranged by MORHAN that aired on national
television in Brazil. Her narrative was a hopeful one, because she felt
that she had resources to draw upon that would help her get through
this difficult phase of her life, and she felt that she also had a purpose
in terms of educating others about leprosy.

Celso

When I interviewed Celso, born in 1954, he was a handsome middle-
aged man with coffee-colored skin who clearly had a good rapport with
the nurses at the public health clinic. He came into the clinic wearing
an Australian bush hat with a Pão de Açucar (the Rio tourist attraction
Sugarloaf Mountain) logo. He used braces to walk; I initially thought
the braces were necessary because of another condition, but his disability was the result of severe nerve damage to his feet and legs from
leprosy. Celso was born in Rio de Janeiro; his mother was from Rio as

well, and his father came from Northeast Brazil. Because of his disability, he had recently been forced to retire from his job as an aviation
aeronautics technician for a Brazilian airline. Celso was married, but
he and his wife were separated; though still living in the same house,
they slept in separate rooms. He had no children. He lived in a working-
class neighborhood not far from the clinic; he characterized the people
in his neighborhood as lower-middle class, "the more humble class,"
who, he believed, were too concerned with what their neighbors were
doing and not interested in larger political or social issues that affected
their lives. I asked if violence was a problem in his neighborhood, and
he responded:

> There's nothing but violence. . . . Drug traffickers, police—I trust
> the traffickers, the *bandidos*, more than the police. Because where
> I live there are more drug traffickers, but they respect me. And
> the police, at least sometimes when I'm getting in my car, some-
> times I'm treated with a lack of respect. I think they are a little
> too aggressive. It's crazy.

His first symptoms of leprosy—pain, swelling, and red spots on
the legs—appeared in 1996. "It hurt and at the same time didn't hurt,
because if you touched them, they were numb. But they hurt a lot."
Although it sounds like a contradiction to say that his legs were painful and numb at once, this juxtaposition seems to occur with many
patients; the pain might be understood as something internal whereas
the surface of the skin was numb to the touch. Celso said there was a
six-month delay between the development of his symptoms and getting
a correct diagnosis of leprosy, during which time his condition rapidly
deteriorated:

> Two years ago—I started to feel it in June. Then I complained to
> the doctor that I'd never felt pain in my legs before. I complained,
> and they said it was varicose veins. Internal varicose veins . . . I
> went around like that until August. . . . I went to a cardiologist.
> I had a lot of pain in my legs and they were very swollen. When
> I got to the cardiologist's, my legs were black, with those purple
> lesions. . . . Then I had a biopsy . . . and from there, there was the

suspicion of hanseníase. From there to here, I suffered a lot. . . .
I stopped walking.

For Celso, leprosy had probably already been attacking his nerves
slowly, but "by the time the spots appeared," he said, "it had already
begun to destroy me, and now I've lost everything—feeling in my fingers, in my hands, in my legs, and I've stopped walking."

When he was diagnosed, he had not heard of hanseníase, but he
had heard of lepra; he was given both terms at diagnosis. "I was scared.
Your arm falls off in pieces, right [*Cai braço em pedaçinhos, né*]? Then,
they gave me some books to read and soon I accepted it." He felt the
term *lepra* was "very depressing. Hanseníase is something more subtle,
you know? Smoother . . . Now lepra is very aggressive. The name, right?"
He was depressed by the diagnosis at first and could not stop thinking
about it: "It didn't leave my head. I cried a lot. I cried and kept crying.
Later, no. Later I got used to the idea and I got more information with
respect to the disease. So, with this information, I got used to it and
adapted. I didn't accept it. I adapted." He also isolated himself, initially.
He anticipated stigmatization from others because of the way some
of the people he knew, particularly those at work, had reacted to the
symptoms, before they knew what disease it was:

> I just hid. First I had to find out if it was contagious. Before find-
> ing out that it wasn't contagious, I just hid. I simply hid. And few
> people know [today] . . . Because, when these blemishes started,
> there were friends of mine who didn't want to touch my hand.
> Friends who used to hug me, kiss me, suddenly distanced them-
> selves from me.

At the same time, he says that since that time, he has not experienced
any stigma directly related to having leprosy—"just from a few friends,
but they did not even know exactly what I had." With his closest friends
(*meus amigos mais chegados*), he also did not reveal his diagnosis, but, he
said, "I think that they knew . . . But they never brought it up with me."

He had come to the conclusion that leprosy was not extremely contagious, because, he said, "If it was, I think that everyone in my family
would have had it. Because I was never separated, not my clothes, not

my bed—nothing was separated. So, I don't think it's contagious, no."
Celso had also reflected on leprosy etiology, and he presented some of
his theories:

> Before this [leprosy] appeared, I was inside a hospital for more
> than two months. I was looking after a cousin of mine who was
> very ill. . . . She was there for surgery . . . and I was with her the
> whole time. She was in a private room, but there were patients
> in isolation, and I'm very curious. I was never afraid. . . . So I
> went to see if these patients needed me. I gave them my hand. I
> wasn't afraid. So it could be from that. And it could also be from
> the type of work I was doing [at the airline]. [There were] several
> chemical agents that were bad—oil, chemical products in gen-
> eral. That could be it too.

Although Celso was given some literature about leprosy at the clinic,
his models of leprosy's etiology and of its transmissibility do not exactly
match the biomedical model. Leprosy is spread from person to person,
but it is unlikely he got leprosy from holding a sick person's hand in
the hospital, since more prolonged contact is probably necessary for
transmission. Exposure to chemicals cannot cause leprosy, though in a
broader sense such exposure might lower immune function, thus theo-
retically increasing susceptibility.

Though Celso had almost finished his MDT regimen when I interviewed him, he was far from being "well," as he was experiencing leprosy
reaction and was at least temporarily disabled. Celso was skeptical that
leprosy was curable; to be cured, for him, would mean a return to the
way life was before he began noticing symptoms. "They have medicines
made for [the symptoms]—creams and pills made in a laboratory, right?
They alleviate; they don't make it better. They don't cure. They work
to alleviate. It makes it possible to live with it." For Celso, side effects
of the medications he was taking were conflated with the symptoms of
leprosy reaction, and he seemed to group all of these problems together
as being "intoxication from medications. But I can't stop taking the
medications," he said, "so I have to live with this intoxication."

Mixed in with skepticism about a full recovery was hope for just that.
Indeed, many of the patients I interviewed did not have a monolithic

view of their future but rather alternated, even within the course of my interview with them, between pessimism and optimism. When I asked Celso the question, "Has leprosy changed your life?" he wavered:

> No, it hasn't changed—yes, it has changed it. I can't say that it hasn't changed it. Because I liked to go to dances, I liked to go out, I liked to travel, to walk. All of these things for me, all of them are over, with this disease. But I intend to return to my life. Walking—I liked to go for walks.

His inability to walk as he used to seemed to be the most devastating transformation in Celso's life. It also inhibited his ability to work:

> I worked up until the end. I worked with a cane and boots. An orthopedic boot. I put it on the right foot because my foot would fall. So while I could stand it, I dragged myself to work. While I could stand it—I had medical leave, but I went . . . I always went to work. And I was doing very badly. When I could, I went. I stopped going when I couldn't walk anymore and [when he got his diagnosis]. Because [then] I went to hide. . . . Later they retired me.

I asked him if he had any special shoes currently, to protect his feet, which could be easily injured because of insensitivity:

> No, I don't know how to get them. . . . I used sandals up until a month ago because sandals are more comfortable. But my feet swell a lot. In a shoe, I can't walk. I put on a shoe and an hour later, I'm in a lot of pain. With tennis shoes, I feel a lot of pain, [my feet] swell more, they squeeze my feet more. . . . The pains persist with the shoes. I don't feel anymore and they get injured. My feet double over, and I lose my balance. It attacks the nerves— neuritis, paresthesia. There doesn't seem to be a cure. I'm not sure, but there doesn't seem to be a cure.

Problems with his legs and feet also limited his mobility. He commented on the difficulty of getting to the health post by bus:

> I come by bus. Until recently I had [a friend] bring me in their car, but I have to gain my independence. I come by bus. It's a bit of

a sacrifice. It's difficult to go up the step, but unfortunately, they
don't . . . think about this. They only think about those who are
healthy, principally here [in Brazil]. In the United States, it's very
different. I was there once . . . I'd like to go back . . . Because there,
the consciousness is very high. . . . Even the bus driver is a humble person. He waits for you to sit, asks you if he can take off.

Although this may not be true for every bus in the United States, certainly the buses in Brazil are not ideal for the disabled. For a person who
does not have full use of his limbs, riding a bus in Brazil can be quite
dangerous. City buses do have a few seats that are larger than others
and with a higher footrest, designed for the elderly and disabled, but
the first step in boarding the bus is a good two to three feet off the
ground and difficult to maneuver with crutches or braces. Although I
noticed that some drivers in Rio wait for elderly or disabled passengers
to find their seats, many buses lurch forward as soon as the last pas-
senger has stepped up onto the first step.

Celso also noted the problems he encountered in trying to maneuver the sidewalks and streets of Rio de Janeiro. Throughout much
of Brazil, sidewalks are constructed of cubes of stone, some cut and
imported from Portugal. These stones are laid together in a mosaic
style, often forming patterns, such as those of the often-photographed
black and white waves on the sidewalks along the beach in Copacabana. Because of the uneven surface of these sidewalks, walking can be
very precarious for those who have any disability of legs or feet. Stones
are often missing or broken, creating even more of a hazard. These
sidewalks are unsafe for walking in general. A Brazilian friend of mine
caught her heel in a hole created by a missing stone and broke her foot.
I was frequently tripped up by these sidewalks, which can be found not
only in Rio but in cities and towns throughout Brazil. Celso said that he
was still capable of walking without braces on a smooth surface, but, he
said, "It's just that on the street, because of the elevations, the holes,
the stones, I lose my equilibrium. I don't trust my legs. Right, left, I
don't feel anything. They're completely numb."

Although not a regular participant in Carnival, he had been invited
to go to the Northeastern city of Recife for the upcoming (1999) Carnival

and was considering the trip. However, because of the problems he has with his feet, he was unsure if he would be able to participate. "People will want to dance. Ah! I'll think about whether I can go . . . I really want to go."

In addition to his feet and legs, Celso believed that his sex drive was affected by the disease and/or its treatment: "I went a long time without—how should I say?—without sexual stimulation. A long time—I think for these two years [since diagnosis]. Now, I'm feeling a little something, you know?" Medication side effects, in addition to his initial self-stigmatization and fear about contaminating others, may play a part in sexual drive and sexual potency. Though his relationship with his wife seemed strained, he did occasionally think about having children: "I had the desire to have children, right? Today, I wouldn't like to have them anymore. First, I think I'm too old. And I don't want to pass it [the disease] to them. I don't know. I'm afraid." I spent some time discussing the biomedical model in which genetic susceptibility may be passed to children, but leprosy itself is not "passed down," that he was no longer contagious at this point anyway.

Celso also said that he had lost "more than 50 percent" of his vision. "I never had problems with my vision [before]." This may have been caused by leprosy, which can damage the ocular nerve, but he had plans to visit an ophthalmologist for the first time the month that I interviewed him, so he did not know for sure. He believed he had incurred minor hearing loss as well. He also believed that he has experienced deterioration in his memory, which he relates to the disease:

CELSO: I believe it's because of the disease because before I didn't have problems with my memory. I wasn't nervous. I was very calm.

C.W.: You think it's worse now, your memory?

CELSO: Much worse. I think it took away a lot of my memory. I can't coordinate ideas. I—mainly, I'm nervous. So I can't coordinate [thoughts] . . . I believe—I'm certain it's connected to the disease because before I didn't have these problems. Now I leave my room to do something, sometimes to go to the bathroom; I leave my room and I've already forgotten what I was going to do.

Celso attributed his perceived memory loss to leprosy, but prednisone is a more likely culprit; this steroid has been cited as a possible cause of memory loss in patients who take it for a prolonged period of time in high doses (Keenan et al. 1996).

Celso had considered suicide, less because of his physical problems than because of the dependency it created. He said that having to depend on others to be able to get around was the most difficult aspect of his life:

> I never depended on anyone for anything, thank God. Since I was
> fourteen, I've been independent. And suddenly I'm dependent
> on the world, right? So this could finish me. Suddenly, I'm in bed
> and I don't have the means to go to the bathroom.

He had managed to overcome thoughts of suicide, however. Religion and his church, he said, provided him with some of the support he needed to move away from suicidal thoughts:

> I think it helps a lot, including in helping people to live because
> thanks to God and to my true friends, who gave me support—I
> thought about committing suicide—human support is also very
> important so that you don't regret doing something stupid.

Celso had recently become a Cristão (evangelical Protestant) though he was searching for his place in that religion:

> Look, before I was nothing, in terms of religion, right? I believed
> that something existed, a God. Today, I'm Cristão. But I'm Cristão
> and not Cristão. I think I am Cristão. I think I am—I consider
> myself normal, because I continue with my ideas. . . . I'm not like
> [those who say], "I'm a better Cristão than you." I'm Cristão, and
> I go to my church often. But I'm still the same person. I continue
> to have my convictions.

My impressions of Celso were that he was an insightful man who was trying his best to seek a cure for his illness, which for him went beyond treating the disease. His primary concern was regaining his independence, which would mean that he would be able to walk comfortably and confidently. Celso was a "good" patient; he sought a diagnosis after experiencing symptoms, never missed an appointment, and always took his medication. He was pleased with the medical services he had received at different health posts where he had been a patient. What could have been done, in Celso's case, to prevent disability? If he had been able to get a diagnosis right away, the problems with his feet and legs may not have been so severe. Special shoes designed for patients with leprosy or diabetes would have been helpful as well; he told me he did not know they existed and did not know how to get them. He had used orthopedic shoes at one point, but they were not made specifically for leprosy patients. Celso should have started physical therapy at the beginning of his treatment. Instead, he had begun just four months prior to my interview with him. He said he waited a long time to start, and now he had started seeing a private doctor for these sessions. Though it is possible that physical therapy would help him regain the use of his legs, the nerve damage that Celso incurred as a result of leprosy and leprosy reaction may affect his mobility permanently or at least require vigilant care of his feet and legs. Still, I had much hope for Celso's future prospects, as he seemed dedicated to doing everything he could (particularly in terms of complying with medical advice and treatment) to get well.

Manoel

A social worker familiar with my project introduced me to Manoel, thirty years old at the time, because his illness experience had been such a difficult one. In addition to suffering from severe leprosy reaction before he had even begun treatment or received a diagnosis, many family members and friends abandoned him during the course of his illness. I chose to include his case because it represents a possible, though perhaps not typical, scenario for leprosy patients in Brazil. I also wanted to illustrate, by recounting Manoel's story, how complex the issue of disease stigma can be.

Manoel was born in 1968 in a suburb of Rio and lived in a low-income neighborhood near the Rio International Airport when I interviewed him. His primary means of making a living, particularly before his condition worsened, was selling items door to door throughout Rio, mainly to people in the favelas: "I go up the hills. I go to Vidigal [a favela at the end of Leblon beach], to Copacabana, to Pavão/Pavãozinho [adjacent favelas on the hills above the Zona Sul neighborhoods of Copacabana and Ipanema]." He preferred selling in the favelas because, he said, "You see a person in a wooden shack, they'll pay the right amount on time, every week. You see a pretty house, a permanent house—they won't pay ten cents." He also traveled to different states occasionally to sell things. He sold a variety of things "for the bathroom, the bed—sheets, towels, cloths . . . a lot of things . . . sometimes even sausage, jerky, cheese. Every day, every week, something different to sell. I get perfume too [to sell]." His work therefore required much walking up the steep hills on which many favelas are built: "I worked going up the hill, down the hill."

In 1995, he noticed a lump or nodule that did not go away. He then started to lose weight rapidly, and he experienced increasing numbness in his feet and legs. Manoel said that while selling door to door, he did not really get enough to eat and also stopped to drink beer frequently, which he felt further exacerbated his symptoms. Soon he could no longer do his job. In addition to having to walk up and down through the favelas, his job required him to carry a heavy bag with his merchandise in it, which became impossible as his condition worsened. During this period of rapid physical deterioration, his wife kicked him out of the house. They had lived together for two years. Her reaction was unrelated to him having leprosy. In fact, his wife had had leprosy in the past. When they split, he was sick, but he had not yet received a diagnosis. He told me first that she and many other family members "disappeared" during that time because they were unsure what he had; they speculated it might be cancer or AIDS. But as our interview continued, he elaborated on other reasons that people abandoned him. The stigma in Manoel's case seemed to derive in part from his drastically changed appearance, weight loss, and visible lesions. He told me that "people were saying things like [they thought] I was going to die. I had lumps [nodules] on my ears, large lumps, my nose bled."

His wife's real motivation for leaving him, however, was that he was no longer able to work or make money once he became very ill, and he attributed having lost some friends to this fact as well. He said that at one point he had a bank account, credit cards, and a car: "When you have money and health, you have a ton of friends. When your situation is broken, your financial situation, you don't have any more friends." He lamented, "People just want material things. Today, no one has love like they used to."

Still, he told me, he continued to have the support and care of his mother. During this time, he said, "I fell asleep crying, I woke up crying, I didn't eat right. . . . My mother would say, 'Calm down, you're going to be all right.' She was very tender with me." Manoel said that in his worse reactional states, he did not have the strength to take a shower and had to use a wash basin with his mother's help. During this time, he said, "People would not get near me. They wouldn't touch me. And when I walked on the street, people avoided me. On a bench, seated on a bench, [people moved away], and I was sitting there alone. . . . No one got near me." Again, people's reactions and stigmatizing behaviors were not a result of them knowing he had leprosy specifically but of his appearance and people's fear of acquiring any disease that appears to be contagious.

He sought medical help and was immediately placed in the hospital, on the grounds of the clinic where I interviewed him; he stayed for fifteen days and was diagnosed with leprosy. "After that, I left, but the numbness and the lumps returned." He began a two-year course of treatment. In addition to numerous episodes of leprosy reaction, he also experienced nausea and loss of appetite from the medications. "I finished treatment [recebi alta] on March 2, 1997," he said. "Now I'm back because I'm experiencing more numbness" from what he called the seqüelas, or scars/lingering effects of the disease. "Because the bacilli stay, right?" he said. I told him they stay but "they're dead." "But the reaction continues," he said. He was back on prednisone for leprosy reaction at the time of the interview.

His illness and the problems it created in his personal life sent Manoel into severe depression. After sessions with a psychologist and a social worker, he was in a better frame of mind, but he told me, "When I had this disease, I tried to kill myself four times. I arrived there at home—my house was under construction—I took a rope, at dawn, and I had my neck in it—but I wasn't able to kill myself." He eventually had the chance to start participating in support groups for leprosy patients, which he found extremely helpful. Manoel expressed his concern that other patients get the psychological help they need so they do not do anything like he did:

> Last week . . . there was a girl here who had hanseníase and also had AIDS. She was expecting a child too. If she didn't have anyone to talk to, she might kill herself because people think that hanseníase has no cure, but it does. It's a very rigorous treatment, but if the person has patience, the person can care for himself. You have to take your medicines, not miss appointments. You always have to come here.

He thought that lectures in which former patients talked to new patients would help people immensely:

> It's good for people to talk to those who already had hanseníase, so that they stay calmer. You say, "I had hanseníase, and many people avoided me." So you give some help to these people, and they are more knowledgeable. "What is hanseníase?" Then you tell them many things, that it's not cancer, it's not AIDS. And people become less desperate. They don't want to kill themselves.

Manoel had clearly spent time considering how leprosy is transmitted. He was aware of many of the popular models of leprosy, and they did not make sense to him:

> Many people say that this disease comes from dogs. If it comes from dogs, what about all the people who have dogs? There are people who have a dog or have a cat in their apartment. . . . There are people who pick up dogs, kiss them on the mouth, kiss dogs, cats. Xuxa [a well-known star of children's television in Brazil] has more than twenty dogs in her house, and she's not sick. So people say a lot of things.

He also commented on the idea that leprosy comes from "the wind":

> AIDS doesn't come from the wind. Cancer also does not come from the wind. So those are two diseases that don't come from

the wind. This disease doesn't come from the wind because [if it did] everyone would be sick.

Instead, Manoel's explanatory model of leprosy etiology more or less mirrored the biomedical model that posits person-to-person contact as the means of transmission. "There are a lot of people with hanseníase in the Baixada; there are a lot in Nova Iguaçu. . . . The buses get full, everyone is sick. No one escapes anything. . . . A person breathes and then these bacilli, they're already there." I heard the same scenario (riding a city bus daily and sharing the same air with people who had leprosy) for possible contagion from healthcare workers at an educational meeting at a clinic in another municipality. However, Manoel's belief in the ease of transmission of leprosy did not match the biomedical model exactly. He suggested, "You have people who leave work, open the fridge, don't wash their hands, pick up a piece of fruit, eat it with the same hand [that had come in contact with an infected person]."

Manoel's life changed in many ways because of leprosy. In addition to not being able to work as he once had, his physical problems prevented him from engaging in other activities he once enjoyed:

> I liked to swim, play soccer. I'm afraid [about swimming] because of the disease, that there wouldn't be anyone to rescue me. . . . One time I went to the beach. I had numbness in my legs. I just swam close to the shore. . . . But there's numbness and then [my legs are] paralyzed, so I was afraid. [People say], "Ah, come play soccer [jogar bola]." Ah, no. I don't play soccer anymore. . . . When you can't do things that you like, you get sort of disgusted.

Manoel was clearly still in the process of making sense of his illness experience. He reasoned, "If a person has to go through this, I think it's written. Because people have to suffer . . . because if you don't suffer, life has no value." He said that he was currently "Spiritist" but was thinking of converting to an evangelical church. "[I'm] just in Espiritismo now. I have a year in Espiritismo. But I'm wanting to return to the church. . . . If I return to the church, it has to be in my heart. . . . I want to be a Cristão. Everybody is. For me to return to the church, I have to have my soul clean."

Manoel was in a hopeful chapter in his own illness narrative when I met him, despite his losses. He was working in odd jobs that he was physically more capable of doing than full-time door-to-door sales, though he preferred being a salesman. When I interviewed him, he was working as a painter for construction jobs, but even that was not easy, and he said he was losing too much weight working at this job. He was still selling when he could; he showed me a brochure with all types of perfumes and creams and natural medicines for which he took orders, both to demonstrate his trade and to see if I had any interest in placing an order. Although he was still experiencing problems with leprosy reaction, he felt that the worst was behind him:

> I was alone. . . . I was abandoned. But I overcame [*venci*]. Many people distanced themselves from me. So, thank God, I was strong. I was brave [*valente*]. I said, "No, I'll overcome this, I'll overcome." And I did.

Elise

The first time I met Elise, she was far too ill to conduct a formal interview with me. She was suffering from a severe leprosy reaction. She had arrived at the clinic in an old car with three of her adult sisters accompanying her, and during her exam, they looked on from outside through an open window and talked with the twenty-three-year-old woman, since there was not enough space in the exam room to accommodate them. As she lay on the exam table, she told me that she had suffered from leprosy reaction since shortly after her treatment began, about a year before. Her brother, who was also treated for leprosy, suffered from reactions, but he was able to take thalidomide. Elise had been prescribed 120 milligrams of prednisone per day at the clinic where she began her treatment. (The World Health Organization does not recommend more than 1mg of prednisone per kilogram of a person's body weight per day; though her weight had increased since beginning prednisone, Elise was well below 120kg, or about 264 pounds.) The referral center where I met her had begun to taper off her dose.

A physician entered the exam room and said that her case was quite complicated. She had been hospitalized for four days at one point; her condition improved while in the hospital but worsened shortly after. Her blood pressure on this occasion was low (90/50), and she had an elevated temperature, so the doctor decided she would need to be hospitalized again. He found an open bed for her at the hospital adjacent to the referral center. I helped her to the car and accompanied her and her sisters to the hospital. She had difficulty walking and was in a great deal of pain, with extremely sensitive skin. Her hospital room was very clean (recently renovated), though not private, and the bathroom was in the hall; another, apparently very ill, patient was already in the room; the hospital treated patients with many ailments, including many patients with AIDS. Elise's sisters asked the staff if they would be allowed to visit her every day, and were told they could.

The following day, one of the physicians at the health post suggested I visit Elise in the hospital to see how she was faring. She was out of her room getting some X-rays, so I did not have a chance to see her. A few months later, I ran into Elise heading up to the health post as I was going to catch a bus. She was in good spirits and walking easily. I told her how happy I was to see how well she looked. Later I was able to sit down and conduct a formal interview with her.

Elise was born in Rio and lived in a working-class neighborhood, Bangu, to the north of the city, a place with violence "like every place has, right?" She went on to explain, "I'm not going to say that it's normal because violence is never normal. It's everywhere, but it's not normal. But you have the bad, violent part and the good part of the community." She lived with her mother and an unmarried sister. She had never been married and had no children. Before being diagnosed with leprosy, she told me she had never been ill. "I never had anything—not even a cold. Everyone would get one and I wouldn't get it. Now with hanseníase, I hardly ever leave the hospital."

Her first symptoms of leprosy, which consisted of swelling in her legs and nodules on her arms and ears, appeared when she was nineteen. She sought diagnosis at a health post close to her home and was diagnosed with leprosy after several tests. She said that she always took her medications and never missed an appointment, but she began to suffer from leprosy reaction from the beginning of her MDT program. Just a few months before, she had been sent to the clinic where I met her because her problems with leprosy reaction required the expert opinions of some of the physicians at this referral center. Now she was taking several medications, including azathioprine, prednisone, and thalidomide. Thalidomide was considered a "last resort" medication for her since it is not supposed to be given to women of reproductive age in Brazil, but she was not currently in a relationship and said she clearly understood the risk of birth defects if she became pregnant.

She thought that she probably got leprosy from her brother, since he was living in the same house with her when he was being treated for the disease. When she learned of her own diagnosis, she already had some knowledge of the disease and its curability based on her brother's experience. His leprosy was a "different type," as she said, so he had an easier time with the disease. Despite the problems she had experienced, she did believe in the curability of leprosy.

Elise was taking university-level courses, but she had to temporarily drop out of school because of repeated episodes of leprosy reaction that resulted in hospitalization:

> I was hospitalized four times. The last time I stayed the longest, which was eighteen days. . . . I had to stop studying. I was in my second year of accounting. . . . Hospitalization, coming and going, coming and going, entering and leaving with reaction. I had a lot of tests [at school]. When I returned from the hospital, I had several tests at the same time, many tests, and lots of material. . . . I was always missing something. . . . I'm going to return this year.

She also felt self-conscious around her classmates when she had visible skin lesions:

> People would ask when they saw my skin this way. It was tiresome. You're making excuses, always lying. . . . I said it was an allergy. But I never said what it really was because I was very afraid of people distancing themselves from me or commenting. This is very tiresome.

Elise did not share her diagnosis with anyone outside of the family. She anticipated that others would stigmatize her because, she said, "Hanseníase is nothing less than the ancient lepra," and she feared that others knew that Hansen's disease and leprosy were the same disease. She recalled a course she took that convinced her that people have erroneous, preconceived ideas about leprosy:

> My teacher brought up the theme of AIDS and of hanseníase. Some people were even saying that hanseníase, even by people in treatment, can be transmitted, which is not true. With the first dose, you cannot transmit it anymore to anyone. So [I thought], "Wow, these people don't understand, don't know."

Of course, such a situation could be seen as an opportunity for her to educate others about the medical model of leprosy, but she equated others' ignorance with potential prejudice against her, so she kept quiet.

Although Elise seemed to have isolated herself from friends and school colleagues, she had a large and supportive family consisting of her mother and a total of eight brothers and sisters, most of whom were married but lived nearby. She also found comfort through her evangelical Protestant church, Assembly of God:

> I go a lot [to church]. I have God as a basis of everything. So, I'm taking my medication, of course, because I have to do my part. But I believe in the power of God, helping me. . . . I do my part so that God can also help me and I get better. I believe in the doctors and in the medication, but above all I believe in God.

At the same time, she did not confide in anyone at her church; she also told people that it was "an allergic sickness and such—I didn't say what it was. Everyone thinks that it was this—an allergy thing."

Elise had not developed any physical disabilities from having leprosy; this may be because she was hospitalized and thus immobile during many of her most severe episodes of leprosy reaction. Her family also had access to a car, and as a student, she did not have to perform manual labor, which can speed up nerve damage to hands and feet. She lived with her family who could help her with household chores.

Elise's story was encouraging in that she believed things would get better for her, and she had periods of relatively good health, as when I interviewed her, which alternated with episodes of fever, pain, and the eruption of new lesions. She planned to resume her studies when she got better. Her treatment regimen for leprosy reaction at the time I interviewed her seemed to be working well for her. However, as she reflected on her experiences with leprosy, she mourned the lost time and the effects the disease has had on her life and self-esteem. "It's changed my life completely, for the worse." She began to cry, then laugh, as I apologized that my questions were making her think too much about everything.

Alexandre

The narrative I will end this chapter with comes from the last interview I conducted during my 1998–1999 fieldwork. I chose to present Alexandre's narrative because it left me optimistic in some ways, and I found it instructive in others. Alexandre, at fifteen, was one of my youngest interview subjects. I had spoken informally with several younger children affected by the disease (with their relatives present), and I had interviewed one thirteen-year-old girl, but her older sister answered most of the questions for her. Often younger people are difficult to interview because they may have trouble articulating their thoughts and expressing their emotions in words. Alexandre proved to be quite mature in terms of his ability to express himself and discuss his illness experience.

Alexandre lived with his parents in a suburb to the north of the city of Rio. His father was a carpenter. He had at one time had four brothers, but two had died accidental deaths. His neighborhood streets were unpaved, and there was no sanitation system, he said. Alexandre came alone to the health post on the day I interviewed him because his father was working and his mother was being treated for a thyroid condition, for which she was to undergo surgery soon. He and his family lived along a river bank on a road where there was high prevalence of disease among the residents, particularly lung diseases, including tuberculosis and "inflamed throat." From the start of his street to his house, he said, "There are sixteen cases of tuberculosis. After passing my house, there are another twenty-five cases. Lots of lung disease." Another health hazard in his neighborhood was created by vehicular traffic. Pedestrian deaths are high in many urban areas of Brazil, particularly in areas where there are no sidewalk overpasses (*passarelas*) over highways or busy roads. He told me that a month earlier, a thirteen-year-old boy, his neighbor, was hit by a car and killed while riding his bike.

Alexandre's first symptom of leprosy, one spot on the skin, appeared when he was eight years old. He had not heard the word *hanseníase* before he was diagnosed, less than a year prior to my interview with him. Before he was diagnosed, he had tried herbs and other home remedies on his skin patches. He said that he was told at his local health post that it could be a skin fungus he got from his dog because he had swum in a pool into which the dog had fallen. Alexandre himself was skeptical, since his dog was sixteen years old and had never been sick. I found it interesting that healthcare personnel had told him his spots might be from contact with a dog, since this constitutes such a popular model of leprosy etiology in Brazil. Alexandre also purchased over-the-counter creams that he bought at the health post pharmacy close to his home. He also tried herbal medicine and "went to church" in attempts to treat his illness. One day, a pharmacist there suspected he might have leprosy; it was this pharmacist who first tested Alexandre's skin patches with a needle for sensitivity and sent him to a treatment center for leprosy the following day.

He received a good orientation about leprosy after he was diagnosed. He said that they gave his mother pamphlets so that she would know more about the disease. He was not sure which form of the disease he had, but he pointed to the blister pack for multibacillary leprosy on a poster. At his church, a branch of the Igreja Universal, they told him that he had a disease that in the past had no cure, and that they killed people who had the disease, but that later a cure was found. Everyone at his church knew about his illness. His teachers and friends at school also were aware that he had leprosy, but this did not seem to affect his status at school. Later on the same day that I interviewed him, he was headed to a performance of a secondary school play of which he was an assistant director; it was organized by his high school but would be presented "on the street" for the people of his community. He seemed enthusiastic about school and about his future. He loved animals and aspired to be a veterinarian.

He had learned the medical model of leprosy etiology, and when I asked him how he thought he got the disease, he said: "What I think— they [healthcare workers] told me that when I was five years old, a person [with leprosy] could have talked with me [thus exposing him to the disease. It started when I was eight. It takes a long time to get like this." His explanatory model reflects the medical model that there is an incubation period of several years for the disease. Although he could not identify exactly where/from whom he got leprosy when he was young, he had since met other people with the disease. He even referred one man to seek treatment: "I sent him here [to the treatment center], but they sent him to do his treatment in the health post [in his town]." Like Manoel and other patients I interviewed, Alexandre's experience with leprosy allowed him to identify symptoms in others and direct them to an appropriate treatment facility. He was faithful in taking his MDT and never missed an appointment.

Alexandre is an example of someone whose life had not been radically changed by the experience of leprosy. Since his diagnosis, his medical care had been excellent, and he told me that his transportation costs were covered by the clinic. He did not experience nerve damage; the only symptoms he had had were spots on the skin. He had only missed school once, since he attended morning sessions; in Brazil, students can choose to attend public school in either morning or afternoon sessions. Though alone at the clinic on the day I interviewed him, he drew on the support of other patients outside the clinic while waiting for his appointments, and he also had a strong support system at home in his family, friends, and fellow churchgoers. Alexandre's narrative suggests the best-case scenario for a person with leprosy from a poor community in urban Brazil. Although individual immune response and perhaps his youth are in part responsible for his physical and emotional resilience, his story also demonstrates the positive outcomes of adequate treatment and support through the enlightened approach and support of community members who seemed to be informed about leprosy and the availability of treatment.

Looking into Lives

The interviews I conducted were open-ended, not only in the sense that the patients I talked with could discuss topics beyond the questions I brought up but also because their stories were all ongoing. Even though some, like Sônia, were "cured," they continued to deal with some of the physical problems associated with leprosy reaction for years afterwards. In the case of Elise and other patients I had the chance to see on multiple occasions, it is evident that changes from one day to the next may be quite drastic for better or worse. Still, as Kleinman notes, though a patient's "life problems keep shifting," the life history "discloses continuities that shape the long-term form of [his or her] illness experience" (1988, 237–238). For most patients, their lives did not pick up again where they had left off before diagnosis but rather changed dramatically as a result of the disease. Not all changes were perceived as negative. Having leprosy, in some cases, gave them a greater sense of compassion and caring toward others; the disease experience provided a purpose to the lives of some patients. However, it was also clear that much of the suffering that these individuals experienced could have been avoided through earlier diagnosis, a simpler treatment program for leprosy and leprosy reaction, and access to better living and employment conditions.

Each time I review my transcriptions of these interviews or listen to the interviewees' voices on tape, I am brought back to the connection these individuals were willing to make with me. Whereas in many traditional anthropological studies, anthropologists have an opportunity to develop close friendships with many of the people in a "community" in which they work, the patients I interviewed came and went, and there were only a few I saw on more than one occasion when they came in for their appointments. Still, I feel that I know many of these people intimately. I found all of the people I interviewed to be incredibly brave and, though some experienced frustration and depression, resilient in facing a difficult illness that was just one part of an already challenging life. By presenting these narratives here and including interview excerpts in previous chapters about the lives of these patients, I have tried to provide some insight into their complex illness experiences. In addition to offering a more holistic portrait of how leprosy affects the daily lives of individuals, these narratives also shed light on some of the ways in which economic and social realities constrain patient agency in their quest to get well.

7

The Final Push?

Patient Agency, Poverty, and Politics

In this book, I have described how leprosy in the contemporary outpatient context affects the lives of several patients in Rio de Janeiro. Some people diagnosed with leprosy sailed through their treatment with relative ease and only minimal disruption to their lives. Others experienced a gamut of physical, social, and economic difficulties as a result of their disease. I have focused on the various problems that patients encounter in finding a diagnosis and completing treatment for leprosy. I have also highlighted, I hope, some of the positive experiences that patients have had in terms of their personal struggle to maintain an optimistic outlook and the support they have received from family and community members as well as from healthcare workers. The patient narratives in chapter 6 demonstrate that these individuals were aware of the stake they have in making sure they get well. They exerted a great deal of effort in seeking treatment and in adhering to the medications, even though they encountered frustration at times. They were also flexible and willing to adopt new cognitive models of leprosy and leprosy treatment, as long as these models matched their experiences. The recognition that patient agency is already being employed by many in Brazil in their efforts to get well is important. Anthropologists Conrad Kottak and Kathryn Kozaitis (2003, 293) assert that human agency "needs only to be activated and expressed" for it to be a powerful force in terms of social change and reform. The majority of patients I formally interviewed or spoke with informally were actors and agents in their paths to wellness, though their agency had not always reached its full expression because of a number of roadblocks they encountered along the way.

The patients I talked to who led me to my conclusions about patient agency may not be representative of all of the people with leprosy in Brazil, or even in Rio de Janeiro. In a sense, they represent the persistent ones, those who did not accept their fate to be ill and took an active role in their treatment. Many also received a great deal of support from people at home, at the health clinic, at church, at work, or in their community. However, we cannot assume that unaccounted-for patients are not also active agents in making decisions about their health. There may be people who tried and temporarily failed (or were let down by the healthcare system) in their quest for a diagnosis and a cure, but their quest may not be complete. All of the patients that I interviewed had been "untreated and undiagnosed" at one time in the past, and some went several years before they received a correct diagnosis. A few patients I interviewed experienced a stage of "denial" about their illness, and one patient abandoned treatment for several months before beginning again.

I would argue that in most cases people want to get well, but the paths they have taken or that are available to them have, for one reason or another, not always been satisfactory. The existence of patient agency in terms of their wellness seeking does not necessarily mean that they are or will be ideal patients. People with leprosy in Brazil may, in some cases, make a decision that the complications associated with leprosy are not significant enough to warrant treatment. Those with the pauci-bacillary form of the disease often experience minor complications; their decision to not seek treatment does not indicate that they do not want to get well but rather that they do not perceive themselves to be sick in the first place. As mentioned in chapter 3, one man, Eugênio, seventy years old at the time of my interview, said he had spots on his back for around twenty years before seeking treatment, assuming they were liver spots associated with aging. Others who actively seek treatment may find that multidrug therapy is difficult to access (in remote areas of Brazil in particular), that clinic visits compromise job time, or that side effects produce distress. In such cases, the decision to abandon or to never seek treatment for leprosy is a logical one from an emic perspective. However, when patients do present themselves at the clinic to seek a diagnosis or begin treatment, the responsibility shifts, at least in part, to the healthcare system to convey information to the patient and provide care that will optimize adherence to medication and reduce the possibility of disability. Nonadherence to treatment is also a significant problem, but it is not necessarily evidence of lack of patient agency in wellness seeking. The most common reasons for nonadherence to treatment in the literature on leprosy in Brazil and elsewhere are related to circumstances in the life of the patient or to aspects of the medical encounter rather than to fatalism or resistance on the part of patients.

Readers of this book who have worked in the medical field may be frustrated with my emphasis on what doctors, nurses, and other healthcare professionals can do in order to make the experience better for patients. Don't patients have some responsibility as well? There are certainly patients who healthcare workers as well as friends and family members might agree are more "difficult" than others. There are patients who do not comply with or who actively resist treatment. There is also a rare, theoretical category of patients with leprosy who become depressed, do not believe they will get well, and want others to be sick. Two people I interviewed (a volunteer and a patient) mentioned this phenomenon. The volunteer told me that some people will think, "Oh, I'm sick? Well, then, everyone else should be sick too." Reports of infecting others with HIV, through attacks with contaminated needles, seem to be rumor-based and related to the insecurity about people with HIV that exists in many societies (Kroeger 2003). However, there are people who have unprotected intercourse when they know they are HIV positive; this documented form of inflicting disease on others has been labeled attempted murder in some countries. With leprosy, a more passive form of "infliction" would take place if a person decided not to undergo MDT knowing that without treatment, he/she might be spreading the disease to others. Even with the forms of resistance to treatment mentioned, one could conceive of interventions that might be useful in getting through to patients who are most resistant to treatment. For example, a person diagnosed with leprosy who "wants everyone else to be sick" because they are sick has most likely not understood that leprosy is a curable disease; they may have embodied notions of leprosy as a disease that transforms a person into a "leper." Through early identification of such attitudes at diagnosis, this problem could be circumvented.

In a recent course I taught on medical anthropology, I optimistically discussed how cultural competency, now a popular catchphrase in public health, can improve patient compliance. A few students asserted that some patients were just "difficult" and that, basically, no amount of persuasion or cultural competency on the part of the physician or family members could help. One student, a nurse herself, told the story of her Caribbean-born grandmother who stubbornly refused to take blood pressure medication every day for the rest of her life, as prescribed by the physician. She was unaccustomed to lifetime treatments, so despite coaxing by her granddaughter and other family members, she would not comply. Another student related that her "full-blooded Cherokee" grandmother refused anything "white medicine" had to offer (which included all aspects of Western biomedicine, regardless of the ethnicity of the practitioners), after a number of negative experiences. An African American student's grandfather refused care from African American physicians, assuming they would not have had the same opportunities and thus skills or education to treat him. Knowledge of patients' perspectives was not enough to change these patients' minds. However, I still believe that there are creative ways, in each case, to make sure patients get well or stay well. Could dietary modifications produce the same effect as daily medication in the woman who did not want to take blood pressure medication for the rest of her life? If the African American man refused to be treated by African American physicians, it seems the family could find another physician who would treat him, if they were not successful in combating his preconceived notions. In respect of the Native American woman, the student revealed that this woman had been healthy her whole life without biomedical care, so in fact it was essentially a nonissue. I am aware, however, from the numerous health crises that have come up in my own family, that illness is a much more complicated experience in its lived context than can be resolved with policy suggestions. Although there are certainly people who might be "irresponsible," in terms of their own healthcare, or "difficult" patients, from the perspective of the healthcare professional, I remain optimistic about the potential of the healthcare worker's role in improving patients' experience with leprosy treatment. This potential is clear from several positive examples I observed at the clinic in Brazil where I spent most of my time. Of course, there are larger structural factors beyond the control of those working in healthcare in Brazil that affect their ability to do their jobs properly, and these, I suggest, are ultimately responsible for the continuation of leprosy in Brazil.

Structural Barriers to Getting Well

At an educational "waiting room" meeting on leprosy I attended at an outpatient clinic, the social worker leading the group introduced me as coming from the United States and asked me to tell the group about the leprosy situation in my country. I said that there were relatively few cases today in the United States, though it had been a problem in the past. A woman spoke up to say, "We wouldn't be here if this was the First World." She saw, correctly, that leprosy was a byproduct of structural violence, where an unequal distribution of wealth, power, and healthcare services, on a global and national scale, negatively affected the health of the poor in Brazil. In his book *Infections and Inequalities*, medical anthropologist and physician Paul Farmer (1999) noted that there are several "constraints" on patient agency in terms of their ability to protect themselves from disease and to comply with treatment. These constraints include wider political, socioeconomic, and historically established forms of inequality that essentially tie the hands of many patients. As Farmer notes, "Calls to change 'lifestyle and behavior' are often directed precisely to those persons whose agency is most constrained" (258).

If we look at leprosy from both an epidemiological and historical perspective, we see that there is a clear correlation between poverty and leprosy. In Europe, leprosy was endemic throughout the Middle Ages; today only the memory of leprosy exists in medieval art and literature and in the structures and cemeteries created for people affected by this disease. Today leprosy can be found primarily in the Southern

Hemisphere though it is not a tropical disease. The Southern hemisphere is where we find most of the developing nations of the world
today, the nations that are most affected by the legacy of European
colonialism and by the current international trends and economic
policies of global capitalism and neoliberalism, which have tended to
concentrate the world's wealth in the hands of a small percentage of
the population and diminish access to resources for the majority of the
world's poor.

Although genetic susceptibility plays a determinant role in why
some people get leprosy and others do not, I think it is important to
consider that poverty and structural inequalities may be the primary
reasons why we still see several hundred thousand new cases of leprosy
each year worldwide. Leprosy is a perfect example of what Paul Farmer
calls, in a chapter title, "biological expressions of social inequalities"
(1999, 262). As the gap between rich and poor nations and individuals
increases, we are going to see an increase in the number of people who
become disabled or die from infectious diseases that are preventable
and/or curable. Social and economic inequities limit not only patient
agency but also the ability of individual healthcare workers in their
efforts to help people get well. Recently, members of the World Health
Organization have started to look at this approach to solving world
health problems. On March 18, 2005, WHO's Commission on Social
Determinants of Health was inaugurated with the goal of addressing the
" 'causes behind the causes of ill health.' " The "social determinants"
they mention are "poverty, social exclusion, inappropriate housing,
shortcomings in safeguarding early childhood development, unsafe
employment conditions, and lack of quality health systems." These factors are broader than the label "social" might imply, but the commission claims to be interested in wanting to "reverse the 'poverty equals
ill-health trend'" (WHO 2005d). The focus seems to be on alleviating
certain aspects of poverty that make it more difficult for the poor to
gain access to health care, though their plans for research include limited reference to concrete changes:

> The Commission will focus the attention of the world's top experts
> and researchers on specific social determinants such as urban

settings, social exclusion, and employment conditions. These "Knowledge Networks" will push the limits of current information to better define the links between social determinants and health, particularly in developing countries. (WHO 2005d)

I believe that the relationship between what they are calling "social determinants" and health has already been established. What, then, can be done to eliminate the root causes of poverty on national and global scales?

As noted in chapter 2, the current socioeconomic reality in Brazil is that millions of people live in shantytown communities in urban areas and millions more live in impoverished conditions in rural areas. There is also a fairly large middle class that nonetheless struggles more than most middle-class Americans do to maintain their economic status. A small percentage of Brazil's population is extremely wealthy. French sociologist Jacques Lambert titled a 1943 book *Os Dois Brasis* (The Two Brazils) in reference to the division that existed between the industrial and wealthy south of Brazil and the impoverished states of the north. While this division between north and south remains, the distinction between the middle/upper classes and the low-income segment of society offers an insight into how two drastically different realities operate simultaneously for different social classes in Brazil. There are numerous structures (in the realms of education, health care, and the criminal justice system, to name a few) in place in Brazilian society that serve to maintain this division. In a footnote to an article that describes the negative consequences for patients and families of the increasing privatization of mental health services in a neoliberal economy, anthropologist João Biehl writes of Brazil that "citizenship has been conceived as universal for the minority rich, regulated according to market inception for the working class and middle class, and denied to poor and marginal multitudes" (2004, 491). Thus, reforms that address this basic division that exists in how citizenship is constructed in Brazil according to social class (which often corresponds to skin color) have the potential to relieve class disparities. There are some programs, such as Favela-Bairro in Rio, that seek to "urbanize" shantytown communities by providing them with basic city services, like sanitation, drinking water, and paved streets. In terms of education, for example, public schools would need to be better funded and would need to provide the type of education, currently available exclusively through private tutoring, that would allow students access to higher education. In terms of health care, a greater percentage of national, state, and local budgets must be dedicated to funding public health services.

Galtung talked about structural violence as often lacking "concrete actors" (1969, 171). In other words, one cannot point the finger at individual people or policies that result in endemic infectious disease, substandard living conditions, and so on. Likewise, it is difficult to find concrete solutions to problems brought about by structural inequalities. In Brazil, a shift would have to take place in the national consciousness regarding the untenable and unjust nature of the class structure for major changes to take place. I would also argue that such a shift must take place on a global level. As global citizens, we must acknowledge that the current socioeconomic disparities among human populations are unacceptable. The consumer model upon which global capitalism is based discourages people across social classes from accepting anything less than that which is available on the market. Thus it becomes difficult to imagine a world where we do not at least aspire to having elite commodities. The money we earn, we begin to think, entitles us to certain luxuries, and any proposal that seeks to redistribute funds through, for example, increased taxation of the middle and upper classes, is perceived as unfair in a capitalistic system that attributes personal success primarily to hard work and ingenuity rather than to preexisting opportunity and advantage on a broader scale. Another shift in human consciousness that is important for all of us is to be able to see people from other ethnicities, social classes, and nations as being intrinsically equal. We should care about poverty and ill health in other countries because the people in those countries are not separate from "us." It is, perhaps, human nature to notice difference, but the construction of "otherness," of difference, as being "less worthy" or "less human" is a social, cultural, and historically mediated phenomenon that we also have the ability, culturally, to overcome.

Because changes in the world system and in the Brazilian socioeconomic structure are not going to be made overnight, we might in the meantime address structural inequalities at the level of patients who are in treatment. Studies with tuberculosis patients (Farmer et al. 1991; Greene 2004) have demonstrated that adherence to complicated treatment programs increases when financial or other types of incentives are offered that alleviate some of the burdens of extreme poverty. The relative success of Sônia's story, detailed in the last chapter, was predicated in part on one of her physicians visiting her at home and bringing her medications both for her symptoms of leprosy reaction and for other health-related conditions that were causing problems for her. Help with the costs of medicines that are not part of the treatment program but that are useful for alleviating medication side effects could enhance patients' trust in the medical system. Transportation coupons for bus or train fare, such as were occasionally but not consistently available to patients when I did my research, could be provided to public health clinics by the federal government/Ministry of Health. These could also be given to family members who accompany patients to the health posts. Identifying and meeting some of the needs that patients have beyond treatment for leprosy can improve patients' experience with illness and could help ensure they complete their treatment regimens.

Targeting the Disease

I will now turn my attention to possible strategies for specific changes that relate to leprosy. What can be done that is not already being done to eliminate leprosy, a curable disease, in Brazil? We might look to strategies that have worked in terms of the elimination of other infectious diseases, such as smallpox and polio (though we are witnessing a reemergence of the latter). Both of these diseases, once a problem worldwide, have been virtually eradicated from even the most impoverished regions of the world through successful vaccination campaigns. Chicken pox, mumps, and measles, once common diseases of childhood, are now virtually unknown.

The BCG (Bacillus Camille-Guerin) vaccine, also used in TB control, offers significant protection against leprosy. When patients were diagnosed with leprosy in the clinic where I spent most of my time, they were asked to bring family members and other household contacts in to receive this vaccine. Vaccination of close contacts of people diagnosed with leprosy, even those who may have received BCG as children (since the effectiveness of the vaccine is believed to diminish over time), is the current policy in Brazil. A study in Malawi that included 121,020 participants demonstrated that revaccination with BCG provided up to 50 percent reduced risk of leprosy (Karonga Prevention Trial Group 1996). A 1999 WHO document on BCG suggests that "the rapid declines of leprosy observed in many countries in Africa have coincided with the wide-scale use of BCG there [intended for TB control], and are consistent with the repeated observation of appreciable BCG protection against leprosy in Africa" (Fine et al. 1999, 26).

Sérgio Cunha, Laura Rodrigues, and Nádia Duppre (2004) note that by the late 1990s, nearly 90 percent of Brazil's infants were receiving the BCG vaccine for tuberculosis control, and in the future, this may translate to a decrease in leprosy incidence. However, these authors write that at present, more needs to be done to prevent the spread of the disease. For revaccination with BCG, they suggest using "a broader definition of contacts" (363), including neighbors and others with whom a patient has close contact. They also suggest the possibility of prevention through chemoprophylaxis, providing MDT drugs to close contacts. Other studies (Nguyen, Cartel, and Grosset 2000; Smith and Smith 2000) have demonstrated correlations between the distribution of single doses of the MDT drug rifampicin and the reduced incidence of leprosy over time. Another possibility in preventing the spread of leprosy among household contacts is the use of new diagnostic techniques to determine who is most at risk for contracting the disease (Cunha, Rodrigues, and Duppre 2004). Bührer-Sékula et al. (2003) describe a test (ML flow test) they developed that can rapidly detect the presence of antibodies to *M. leprae*; these antibodies indicate not only that a person has been exposed to the disease but also that they are likely to develop multibacillary leprosy in the future, though clinical signs have not yet manifested. This would be promising for people who have spent significant amounts of time with a person who has been diagnosed with leprosy. Expanding the number of contacts that are brought in for BCG revaccination, for chemoprophylaxis, or for diagnostic testing does increase the risk of stigma for the patient, however, since it requires notifying more people in a patient's circle of acquaintances about his or her illness, so care would have to be taken in this regard.

The development of an effective shorter-term MDT program would be helpful in terms of eliminating some of the problems associated with adherence, but clinical trials would be necessary to ensure that shorter treatment regimens would not involve problems with relapse. Lockwood and Kumar (2004) have suggested that there is not enough data on relapse rates to support WHO's decision to decrease the treatment time for multibacillary patients from twenty-four to twelve months. When I was in Brazil, testing had recently begun on a single-dose treatment called ROM, an acronym for the three drugs of which it consists (rifampicin, ofloxacin, and minocycline) (WHO 1999). However, only patients with paucibacillary leprosy who have a single lesion were eligible. Children are excluded altogether because ROM can stunt their growth, and minocycline (a tetracycline) can cause dental problems in children (Talhari and Neves 1997). Shortened treatment programs would be ideal for patients, but the risk of relapse and leprosy reaction must be considered in implementing changes to MDT.

I turn my attention now to what might be done, and what is being done, in Brazil, to improve leprosy control. Early detection is the key, I believe, to both controlling the spread of the disease and preventing disability. Because most cases of leprosy are not difficult to detect, a yearly screening in the public schools could be very useful in the elimination of the disease. Such an early detection program would not have to be inordinately expensive, as it is simple to train volunteers or teachers to determine if a lesion or spot on a person's body is insensitive. Of course, there are potential problems with such a screening system. First of all, there is no way to ensure that an individual will actually go to a health post if he or she is suspected of having leprosy. Second, and perhaps more important, is the fact that leprosy stigma still exists in Brazil, and a diagnosis or even suspicion of leprosy could prompt school officials to restrict a child's access to school. Although such exclusion is illegal, it does occur, as with one of the patients I interviewed (Odete, age thirteen), who was temporarily not allowed to attend her school because of her illness. Leprosy screening programs would have to be accompanied by educational programs about the disease for both parents and teachers at schools if such a program were to be successful. Ideally, such a screening program could also detect other skin diseases among children. Teachers I spoke with at a public school adjacent to a favela told me that many of their children suffer from scabies, funguses, rashes, and other skin ailments that go untreated.

Mandatory training in detecting leprosy in its early stages should be a part of all medical school curricula in Brazil, and physicians working in both private practice and the public health system should learn to think of leprosy as a possibility in any case where numbness, visible skin changes, or nerve problems are present. Media campaigns about leprosy, many of which are already in place and are discussed in more detail below, also have great potential in terms of increasing awareness of early symptoms of leprosy. For patients in treatment, more information and careful explanation by healthcare workers of what patients might expect, in terms of potential side effects of medication and leprosy reaction, could play a part in ensuring patient compliance and trust in the biomedical system and in improving patient experience. It is also important for healthcare workers to have a clear understanding of the everyday realities of the living and working conditions of the patients they treat, as these realities can impact the treatment program and the instructions that patients are given for caring for their hands and feet and for taking MDT at home.

Increased access to leprosy treatment is another aspect of improved detection rates that the Brazilian Ministry of Health is taking into account. The process of decentralization of leprosy services through "municipalization"—making municipalities, or cities, responsible for leprosy treatment and, ultimately, having MDT blister packs available at all public health clinics—started in 1998, the year I began my research. Decentralization has potential in terms of giving patients more options for treatment locations. A disadvantage is that local governments are put in charge of medication distribution and funding to public health posts, so that care may be compromised in municipalities where funds are not properly managed. Another concern is that patients who go to regular health posts once a month to pick up their treatment will not receive the kind of expert care that is available at treatment centers that are specifically for leprosy care, like those where I conducted most of my observations. Disability prevention might thus be compromised. However, the wider coverage with MDT might outweigh the disadvantages of the decentralization plan. Prevalence rates have indeed dropped significantly—from 79,908 total cases (4.6 per 10,000) registered at the beginning of 2004 to 30,603 cases (1.7 per 10,000) at the beginning of 2005—(WHO 2005a), though I suspect this may be related to changes in case reporting, a factor that will be discussed further below.

There are two arenas of human interaction in Brazil that may impact leprosy control efforts that I would like to touch upon briefly—the armed services and the prison system. Two years of military service is "mandatory" for men in Brazil, though most middle- and upper-class men are able to receive deferments, so "as a result the ranks are made up primarily of lower-class and lower-middle-class recruits" (Country-data.com 1997). A few of the patients I met and interviewed who had been treated by army or navy physicians (and later referred to the leprosy treatment center where I worked) had been placed in isolation during treatment, and at least one mentioned being treated with a medication that dates back to pre-MDT treatment. I do not know whether military healthcare personnel in Brazil are now up-to-date in their treatment and care of people affected by leprosy, but if not, this is a significant area of public health concern, particularly because the conditions of military living, in military barracks, contribute to the spread of airborne bacilli. Even more urgent in terms of leprosy control and public health is the situation in Brazilian prisons. As with the military and so many other areas of Brazilian life, there are essentially separate prison privileges for the middle/upper classes and the lower class. Since 1941, Brazilians who have a university degree, as well as government officials, highly ranked officers of the armed forces, police chiefs, and other individuals in positions of relative power have been accorded the privilege of *prisão especial*. "Special" inmates "must have 'adequate' quarters, unlimited access to legal assistance, unrestricted visits from friends and relatives, uncensored mail, religious assistance when possible and medical assistance when necessary" (Altieri 2001, 18). Meanwhile, the conditions for prisoners who come from impoverished backgrounds, have been described as horrific by numerous human rights organizations and officials. In the documentary *Bus 174* (*Ônibus 174*) (Padilha and Lacerda 2002), about a city bus held hostage in Rio de Janeiro by a man who grew up on the streets and spent time in prison in Brazil, the filmmakers visited and filmed in one of the prisons in Rio. One man interviewed in the prison said that he had leprosy (using the word *hanseníase*) and was not receiving treatment for it. I cannot speculate on whether this statement was true, but the organization Human Rights Watch, in a 1998 report, noted that prisoners with TB and HIV were not receiving proper treatment in Brazil (Mariner and Cavallaro 1998), while at the same time prison conditions foster the spread of these diseases and the exacerbation of symptoms. Like TB, the leprosy bacillus is especially amenable to prison life because it is spread through droplets emitted during breathing. Though prison reform may be moving at a slow pace in Brazil, the Ministry of Health should at the least ensure that leprosy diagnosis and especially treatment of previously diagnosed cases takes place in the prisons.

Leprosy Education, Social Marketing, and the Media

Education is one of the more important parts of leprosy control. I saw many examples of the effectiveness of MORHAN's leprosy-education campaigns. During lectures, puppet shows, and presentations about leprosy given in Rio de Janeiro, there would usually be at least one individual in the audience who had symptoms and was referred to a health post. I witnessed this twice when I accompanied MORHAN volunteers to public schools. MORHAN volunteers told me that at one lecture they gave in the *favela* of Vigário Geral in Rio, there were approximately twenty-five participants, and among them, ten presented suspect symptoms of leprosy. Children are an especially good audience for leprosy-education campaigns, they said, because they usually have no preconceived ideas about the disease. Three MORHAN volunteers told me (in separate interviews) their versions of the following story, which illustrates how successful their educational work with children is:

> We went to a school in Nova Iguaçu and performed our puppet show, and a child identified a spot on his arm that looked like

the spot on the doll. So, he asked his mother to take him to the doctor. She took him, and they found that he had hanseníase. His mother cried a lot. He took her into the [MORHAN branch, adjacent to the health post in Nova Iguaçu], and he said, "Miss, I came to get a note for school." And we were able to get this boy to calm his mother down, to calm down his family, and now, he participates to help others learn. It was very beautiful. Very good.

The volunteers were impressed by this boy who had no fear of the disease. He knew only what he heard at school, which is that with treatment, hanseníase is curable. Children, the MORHAN volunteers said, have not yet learned the stigma of leprosy or of disease in general and thus do not hesitate to diagnose themselves or other family members if they find an insensitive spot that resembles what was described in the puppet show.

Media campaigns are also vital in getting information about leprosy to a wide audience. Care must be taken in how messages about leprosy are "marketed." As Mee Lian Wong (2002, 314) astutely wrote, "Selling the message on 'cure for leprosy' is not like selling soap or chocolates. The 'product' that is promoted in leprosy health education—is often intangible and offers gratification in the often distant future." One form of social marketing used by MORHAN and by the Ministry of Health is the production of educational posters and fliers. MORHAN volunteers conduct *panfletagens*, or distributions of informational pamphlets about leprosy. These pamphlets contain information about the symptoms and treatment of the disease, MORHAN's phone number, and addresses for health posts in Rio de Janeiro that offer Hansen's disease treatment. Posters are also a useful way to disseminate information about leprosy. Four patients I interviewed formally (out of nineteen who had heard the word *hanseníase* prior to diagnosis) said that they knew about it from posters they had seen. One (Janete, age forty-one) said that seeing these posters allowed her to identify her symptoms and seek treatment at a health post. In Telehansen phone calls, several people had seen posters, fliers, or pamphlets with information on leprosy and with MORHAN's phone number. I saw some of MORHAN's posters on public buses in Rio, which is an excellent location, since thousands of people see them every day. These posters also appear in health posts in some parts of the city.

The main poster that was in use when I was in Brazil was one with photos of a man's face "before multidrug therapy" and "after multidrug therapy." In the "before" photo, the man's face is swollen and covered with nodules from large concentrations of bacilli. In the "after" picture, the man's face looks relatively normal, with only minor evidence (like acne scars) that he ever had a problem. However, according to Artur Custódio de Sousa of MORHAN, this poster was not popular among patients because they feared that they would become like the man in the "before" photo, which represents an extreme case of multibacillary leprosy. The "after" photo, which demonstrates the effectiveness of multidrug therapy, was thus overshadowed by the frightening "before" image.

A more recent series of posters that were being produced in the late summer of 1999, shortly before I completed my fieldwork in Brazil, presented a more positive image, or, as acknowledged by MORHAN, an image appealing to aesthetic sensibilities. These posters show healthy, attractive individuals, such as, in one poster, a little girl, and the words, "Would you say that I had Hansen's disease?" (*Você diria que eu tive hanseníase?*) There is also information on the poster about the treatment and the cure for leprosy. Each poster features individuals about whom no one would suspect that they had already been treated for a serious disease. The aim of this series of posters is to reduce stigma and to show that with treatment, one can look "normal."

However, posters that show examples of the lesions associated with leprosy may be more effective in terms of helping patients to self-diagnose. Gerson, twenty-three, thought it was good to have posters in prominent locations because "sometimes people have symptoms but don't know what it is. So, looking at the posters, at the propaganda, they might . . . come in to be treated. This is very good. The posters orient people. They're good for explaining." Nelson, twenty-eight, agreed:

> I think people are well-informed because there are many informational posters in the health posts of the Baixada. . . . I went to the health post. It's written there, "Hansen's disease is curable"

Leprosy-awareness poster focusing on the curability of the disease and on the idea that the disease does not have to be disfiguring. The poster reads, "Would you say that I had leprosy?" Photograph of poster by Cassandra White.

[*Hanseníase tem cura.*] And it says about the spots on the skin—I think people are better informed.

Television in particular is an important way through which the Ministry of Health could improve early detection. Two patients I formally interviewed (of the nineteen patients who had heard the term hanseníase before diagnosis) said they knew about the disease from television. Another patient, Regina, thirty-four, said that she started noticing public service announcements about hanseníase after her diagnosis. Laura, a patient in her forties, remembered hearing on television, "When you see a little spot [*uma manchinha*], go to the nearest health post." She said she had detected a small lesion that was numb, and that the television campaign played a part in her seeking treatment. More frequent use of the media to increase awareness of leprosy and its symptoms would be an important way to increase detection of new cases.

Celebrity involvement is another social-marketing tool that has been shown to be useful with many illnesses. MORHAN has been fairly successful in recruiting Brazilian celebrities and well-known personalities into their movement. In 1988 soccer star Pelé lent his name to the cause of leprosy awareness, although he is no longer involved. In 1999 MORHAN began working on leprosy education with Rosinha Garotinho, who was at the time married to Rio de Janeiro's governor, Antônio Garotinho but later served as governor herself. Singer Ney Matogrosso and actress Solange Couto are active spokespeople for MORHAN today. MORHAN has yet to find a single celebrity who has had leprosy, though Couto has been personally affected by the disease. She became involved with MORHAN after Ney Matogrosso made a guest appearance and talked about leprosy on *The Clone*, a very popular 2002 novela. Solange Couto was a speaker at the International Leprosy Congress in Salvador, Brazil, in August 2002. She entered the enormous conference room, which was overflowing with people, many of whom had to sit on the floor, followed by a news crew, and she was showered with applause and flower bouquets. She told the audience, composed of leprosy researchers, NGO volunteers (including many former patients), and local media representatives, that her mother had the disease and had been treated for it. She also recounted her personal experience of weight gain associated with prednisone, which she took for allergies. She talked about how stigmatizing carrying extra weight could be in Brazil, and how she was denied acting jobs because of it.

Novelas have perhaps the greatest potential for disseminating public health information in Brazil today. Response to public health information that is intricately woven into novela storylines is well documented. For example, the 2000 Brazilian novela *Laços da Família* (Family Ties) featured a character with leukemia who needed a bone marrow transplant; blood donations and registration of potential bone marrow donors both went up significantly while the novela aired (Andaló 2003). The president of the organization Population Media Center, which funds and facilitates the incorporation of public health messages into serial television dramas in developing nations, cites a number of similar examples of the effectiveness of such campaigns (Ryerson 2005). The incorporation of public health messages about leprosy into one episode of *The Clone* may have had some impact on awareness, but I believe that if a character affected by leprosy were made central to the plot of a Brazilian novela, it would do wonders for leprosy detection and treatment.

Global Politics and Leprosy

Since the introduction of multidrug therapy treatment for leprosy in the 1980s, it has become more possible to imagine a world without this disease. By 1991 the prevalence of leprosy had dropped so dramatically that WHO representatives felt comfortable announcing a goal to eliminate leprosy by the year 2000. "Elimination" refers to the reduction of total number of cases to one per ten thousand people in a given region. However, in 1991, elimination was an unrealistic goal in many endemic nations. Although prevalence seemed to be decreasing, the number of new cases of the disease was not (though it has begun to drop since 2000). In addition, the way in which WHO calculates leprosy prevalence indicates that statistics on prevalence may not reflect the reality. Feenstra (2003, 250) points out that WHO's calculations of prevalence were flawed because they were subject to changes in the duration of the treatment program and "updating of the registers ('cleaning' of the registers has contributed tremendously to the decline, which in some countries was sufficient to 'eliminate' leprosy)." "Cleaning" refers to dropping patients who have abandoned treatment from official registers after twelve months though they have not completed their treatment and may still be actively transmitting leprosy, as discussed in chapter 4.

The theory behind elimination is that reducing prevalence to one case per ten thousand will naturally result in eradication. S. K. Nordeen, the director of the Leprosy Control Programme at WHO at the time, commented, "The chances of leprosy staging a comeback at that point are unbelievably small. . . . At a certain point, it is likely the disease will not be able to survive" (quoted in Hassel 1997, A-8). Many disagreed with Nordeen's position. Dr. Paul Brand, formerly of Carville, commented at the 1993 International Leprosy Congress that the elimination campaign was a dangerous one. In the 1940s, he said, they were equally optimistic that sulfones would eliminate leprosy from the world: "Those were exciting times, and many people were convinced that dapsone would rid the world of leprosy within a generation. . . . Of course, it didn't happen. The disease developed resistance, and here we are, still living in a world where small children can contract leprosy and go years, even a lifetime, without treatment" (quoted in Hassel 1997, A-8). Brand was concerned that people would stop thinking about leprosy as a problem, and funds for leprosy research would disappear. According to a social worker I interviewed in Brazil, this is exactly what came to pass. After this goal was announced, she said,

> There was a real retreat, a reduction of resources from international organizations. . . . [It was said that] leprosy would be gone and that these international organizations would have to begin work on other fronts. . . . There was a very large cut here . . . from professionals to the maintenance of shoe shops and materials. . . . For ten years, SERFA [an organization associated with American Leprosy Missions] had great coverage in preventing disabilities. They gave educational courses. So all of this diminished.

More recently, Dr. David Scollard, editor of the *International Journal of Leprosy and Other Mycobacterial Diseases*, commented that "the perception that the elimination of leprosy is imminent has undoubtedly discouraged many scientists and funding sources from pursuing it further" (2005, 26), even though much is still not known about how the leprosy bacillus operates in the human body.

In 1999 WHO created the Global Alliance for the Elimination of Leprosy (GAEL) for another "final push" to attempt to eliminate leprosy by 2005, which was a goal that was not met in many endemic regions. In addition to WHO, GAEL members included Ministries of Health in endemic nations and several organizations that provide major sponsorship for leprosy treatment and research (Skolnik et al. 2003). ILEP (the International Federation of Anti-Leprosy Associations), which included many nonprofit organizations that fund leprosy work, was initially a member of GAEL but was expelled after disagreements about policy.

A Turning Point?

After some criticism of GAEL and of WHO's policies from within the international community of leprosy organizations and scholars, WHO officials have decided to "discontinue the campaign approach" (WHO 2005b, v). This decision was surely influenced by an evaluation of GAEL (Skolnik et al. 2003) that was based in part on interviews with one hundred informants worldwide who have extensive experience in leprosy work. This report noted concerns among workers in the field about the value and "validity" of data on incidence and prevalence of leprosy, particularly "in the face of operational factors such as change in case definition of the disease, duration of treatment, and criteria of cure" (Skolnik et al. 2003, 8). The authors of this independent evaluation encouraged greater collaboration with existing NGOs, and they suggested an "explicitly broad-based approach to the control of leprosy, the avoidance of nerve damage, and the rehabilitation of those in need" (Skolnik et al. 2003, 20).

A recent document produced by WHO, "Global Strategy for Further Reducing the Leprosy Burden and Sustaining Leprosy Control Activities," reflects positive changes in policy:

> In view of the need to sustain leprosy services for many years to
> come, there has been a shift from a campaign-like elimination

approach towards the long-term process of sustaining integrated, high-quality leprosy services which, in addition to case detection and treatment with multidrug therapy, also include prevention of disability and rehabilitation. (WHO 2005b, 2)

This document reflects a shift that addresses several of the problems that are related to the treatment program as I observed it in Brazil in 1998–1999. The new policy, at least on paper, presents a more holistic vision of patient care than previous policies that seemed to focus more on "elimination":

One frequently neglected aspect is the provision of services for long-term care of patients suffering from the sequelae of nerve damage, for example chronic foot ulcers and leprosy reactions. These will need, besides medical and surgical interventions, support from proper counselling services. (2005b, 13)

Interventions [should be] aimed at preventing disabilities/impairments from occurring and/or worsening including early detection and effective management of leprosy-related reactions and nerve damage. (WHO 2005b, 13)

The Global Strategy will need input from ongoing and future research studies being conducted globally, in order to improve the quality and quantity of the tools and procedures available for leprosy control. The priority areas for research are prevention and management of nerve-function impairment and reactions, improving chemotherapy, developing and improving diagnostics to identify individuals in the community who are at high risk of developing leprosy and operational research to improve the sustainability and integration of leprosy services. (WHO 2005b, 13)

I am optimistic about the possibility of eradicating leprosy in Brazil and in the rest of the world, but I believe that there is much still to be done to reach this goal and that it is at least a generation away from taking place. Although the focus of my research was on the level of the people directly affected by leprosy, I hope I have been able to convey, at least in part, the complexity of the task of leprosy eradication and the relationship of leprosy-control efforts to international policies and political and economic forces. There is still a high risk that, if "elimination" is settled for and the global health community turns its attention away from leprosy, this disease, one of the oldest known to humankind, will never disappear.

APPENDIX A:
INTERVIEW QUESTIONS FOR PATIENTS

Below are the questions that I used to gather illness narratives from people in different stages of treatment for leprosy in Rio de Janeiro. Although I attempted to ask each participant all of the questions included here, I also allowed patients to talk about topics that were not covered in my interview schedule. In some cases, I followed up with new questions based on participant responses. I asked native speakers to check my Portuguese before beginning my interviews, but in retrospect, some of the phrasing I used at the time was awkward. In some cases, I would rephrase questions on the spot if participants were unclear with what I was attempting to ask. While I use the term "*você*" (you, casual) in this text of my interview, I used the more formal or polite terms for "you"—"*o senhor*" and "*a senhora*"—in many interviews, particularly when the interview subject was older than me. In Brazilian Portuguese, *tu* is used only in intimate relationships or close friendships.

What is your date of birth?
Qual é o dia (a data) do seu nascimento? Em que ano?

Where were you born?
Onde você nasceu?

Could you talk a little bit about your parents (where they are from, what they do/did for a living)?
Você podia falar um pouco sobre seus pais (de onde eles vieram, em que eles trabalharam)?

Do you work/what do you do for a living?
Em que você trabalha agora?

Could you talk about your childhood? Where did you grow up? Did you have brothers and sisters? Did you go to school? Did you work?
Podemos falar de sua juventude?: Onde foi criada? Teve/tem irmãs e irmãos? Foi à escola? Trabalhou?

Do you have children? How many? Are you married/live with someone? Who are the members of your household at present?
Você tem filhos/ quantos? Você está casado/moram juntos? Quem são os membros do seu lar agora?

How old were you when you first had symptoms of Hansen's disease? What were the symptoms? Did you recognize these symptoms as Hansen's disease at first or did you associate them with another illness?

Quantos anos você tinha quando apareceram os primeiros sintomas de hanseníase?
Quais eram as sintomas? Você reconheceu estes sintomas com hanseníase ao
princípio ou é que pensou que tinham a ver com outra doença?

Did anyone else in your family or community have Hansen's disease?
Houve outra pessoa na sua família ou comunidade que tinha hanseníase?

How do you think you got the disease?
Como você acha que pegou a doença?

Had you hear the word Hansen's disease before? The word leprosy? How
much did you know about the disease before you contracted it?
Já ouviu a palavra "hanseníase" antes de contratá-lo? a palavra "lepra"? Sabia
algo da doença antes de pegá-lo?

When were you diagnosed with Hansen's disease? Who diagnosed you?
How did you respond to the diagnosis?
Quando foi diagnosticado com hanseníase? Quem lhe deu a diagnose? Como
respondeu à diagnose?

If you were diagnosed by a physician or nurse, did you receive any educational materials to take home when you were diagnosed?
Se você fosse diagnosticado por um médico ou uma enfermeira, você recebeu algu-
mas matérias educacionais sobre hanseníase para levar à casa?

Did you have any preconceived ideas about the disease?
Antes de contratá-lo, teve alguns preconceitos sobre esta doença?

What do you think are the causes of Hansen's disease?
Que pensa você sobre as causas de hanseníase?

Did you tell your family/friends/people at work about the disease? If so,
what was their reaction?
Você falou com sua família sobre a doença?
Falou com os amigos?
Com as pessoas no trabalho?
Se a resposta for "sim," quais foram suas reações?

[If you kept it a secret] how did you conceal the disease from others?
[Se não divulgasse] como escondeu a doença de outras pessoas?

Have you experienced stigma related to Hansen's disease at home/ at
work/ in the community?
Você foi estigmatizado (experimentou preconceitos) alguma vez no trabalho, na
casa, ou na comunidade por causa de ter hanseníase?

Has your family experienced stigma because of your disease?
Alguma vez você foi estigmatizado (havia preconceitos contra) sua família por
causa de sua doença?

Do you know what form of the disease you have?
Sabe qual tipo de hanseníase tem?

Were you tested by a physician for Hansen's disease? Do you know what
test they used?

Foi examinado por um médico para detectar hanseníase? Sabe quais métodos foram usados? Qual era a prova/teste usada?

Are you currently taking medications for Hansen's disease? What medications?
Você está tomando medicamentos para hanseníase agora? Quais são?

Do you feel these medications have been effective in clearing up your symptoms?
Você sente que estes medicamentos têm sido efetivos contra seus sintomas?

Are you allergic to any of the medications used in multidrug therapy?
Você tem alergias a uns dos medicamentos na quimoterapia da hanseníase?

Have you experienced any side effects from these medications? What are some of the more severe side effects you have experienced from Hansen's disease medications?
Você experimentou efeitos colaterais/ complicações destes medicamentos? Quais são algumas das complicações severas que você tinha dos medicamentos contra hanseníase?

Have you ever had to stay home from work because of side effects from the multidrug therapy?
Você as vezes tem que faltar dias de trabalho por causa dos efeitos colaterais/ complicações da poliquimioterapia?]

Have you tried any alternative treatments (or home remedies) for Hansen's disease (treatments recommended by friends/family or specialists in the community)? Have you tried alternative treatments for other diseases or illnesses?
Você tentou alguns tratamentos alternativos (ou remédios caseiros) por hanseníase (tratamentos pela recomendação de companheiros/família ou de especialistas locais)? Tentou tratamentos alternativos para outras doenças?
(I found that I did not elicit the expected response from the above question. Eventually, I found out that if I rephrased the question, using the words "remédios caseiros" (home remedies) instead of "tratamentos alternativos," I began to get a better response.)

Do you ever buy medications at the pharmacy to help you with the symptoms of Hansen's disease? With pain?
Você as vezes compra medicamentos da farmácia para lhe ajudar com os sintomas de Hanseníase? por dores gerais?

What is your faith (Catholicism, Protestantism, Umbanda, Candomblé, Macumba, Spiritism, other, combination)?
Qual é sua fé (Catolicismo, Protestantismo, Umbanda, Candomblé, Macumba, Espiritismo, outra, uma combinação)?

What church services do you attend if any?
Você assiste serviços religiosos de alguma forma?

How does your faith help you deal with having Hansen's disease?
Como sua fé lhe ajuda enfrentando o dia a dia com hanseníase?

Where do you go for treatment? Do you go to one or more clinic?
Onde você vai para seu tratamento? Vai a mais de uma clínica por hanseníase?

How many times do you go to the clinic/health post each month (for Hansen's disease-related treatment/problems)?
Quantas vezes por mês você vai à clínica/pôsto de saúde (por problemas com o tratamento ou relacionados à hanseníase)?

Do you like the doctors at the health post/ clinic? Are you comfortable discussing with them your illness and the problems associated with it?
Você gosta dos médicos no posto de saúde/ na clínica? Você sente cômoda falando com eles sobre sua doença e os relacionados problemas?

Do you have confidence in your physicians at the Hansen's disease clinic?
Você confia nos seus médicos na clínica de hanseníase?

What has your experience been with doctors/nurses at other health posts or hospitals?
Como foi sua experiência com médcios/enfermeiras de outros postos de saúde ou hospitais?

How do you get to the health post/clinic?
Como você chega ao pôsto de saúde?

Have you ever missed an appointment? Why?
Você alguma vez faltou de ir à clínica no dia marcado? Porque?

Do you have to miss work to visit the health post/clinic? If so, what repercussions does missing work have for you?
Você tem que faltar o trabalho para ir ao posto de saúde/à clínica? Se a resposta for "sim," quais são as conseqüências de faltar um dia de trabalho?

[If applicable]: Do you have to find someone to take care of your children when you go to the clinic?
[Se for relevante]: Você tem que conseguir alguém para cuidar dos seus filhos quando vai à clínica?

Have you ever discontinued your medications? Why? Did discontinuing your treatment result in a return of any of your symptoms?
Você alguma vez parou de tomar seus medicamentos para hanseníase? Porque? Voltou alguns sintomas depois que você parou com o tratamento?

Have you ever taken medications given to you by someone else with Hansen's
disease (medications not prescribed directly to you)?
Você alguma vez tomou medicamentos que outra pessoa com hanseníase conseguiu e lhe deu a você?

Do have any disabilities you associate with Hansen's disease (complications with hands and feet, eyesight, infection, amputation)?
Você tem alguma deficiência física que você liga a sua hanseníase (complicações com as mãos ou os pés, problemas com os olhos, infecções, amputação)?

Have you been instructed to take special precautions to prevent disability of hands or feet?
Foi instruído por um médico tomar precauções especiais para prevenir problemas com as mãos ou os pés?

Were you ever given any special equipment to protect you from disabilities caused by insensitivity in hands and feet (e.g., special shoes)?
Foi dado algo para lhe proteger de incapacidades causadas por maõs e pés insensíveis (por exemplo, sapatos especiais)?

Do you receive a pension from the government because of this disease? Did you have to apply for this pension yourself?
Você recebe uma pensão do governo por causa desta doença? Teve que fazer uma solicitação por esta pensão?

Besides Hansen's disease, do you have any other health problems?
Além de hanseníase, você tem outros problemas com a saúde?

What is your opinion about contagion with regard to Hansen's disease?
Pode falar de sua opinião sobre contágio com respeito à hanseníase?

Do people in your community think of this disease as contagious?
As pessoas na sua comunidade pensam que esta doença seja infecciosa/contagiosa?

How do you feel about the word *leprosy* as opposed to *Hansen's disease*? *Leper?*
O que você pensa sobre a palavra hanseníase *em relação à palavra* lepra? Leproso?

Do you tell people you have leprosy or Hansen's disease [if you tell them anything]? How do they react?
Você fala que tem "lepra" ou "hanseníase" [se fale algo]? Como reacionam?

In what ways has having Hansen's disease changed your life?
Como mudou sua vida ter hanseníase?

Has it affected your decisions about whether to have children/ more children? Why?
É que sua enfermedade afeitou suas decisões de ter filhos/mais filhos? Porque?

Do you ever forget you have Hansen's disease?
Você as vezes esquece que tem hanseníase?

Some general questions:

Do you enjoy living in Rio de Janeiro in comparison with other cities [for those who have migrated]?
Você gosta de morar aqui no Rio em comparação com outras cidades [para as pessoas que são migrantes]?

What is it like where you live? (urbanized with paved streets, sanitation? favela-bairro? favela? apartment or house?)
Como é sua comunidade? (urbanizado? saneamento? favela-bairro? favela?)

Have you found opportunities for work here?
Você achou bastante oportunidades para trabalho aqui?

Do you participate in community activities? Work groups?
Você participa em atividades comunitárias? mutirões?

Are you a member of a samba school? Do you participate in Carnival?
Você é um membro de uma escola de samba? Participa no Carnaval?

Do you participate in politics—election campaigns, local offices?
Você participa em coisas políticas, no nível local—campanhas eleitorais, cargos
    políticos locais?

What issues do you feel are most important to people in this community?
Quais são os assuntos mais importantes às pessoas aqui nesta comunidade?

Do you feel this community is united?
Você acha esta comunidade unida?

What are the greatest difficulties you face on a day-to-day basis? [If Han-
    sen's disease is the answer, then]: Aside from Hansen's disease?
Quais são as dificuldades maiores que você encontra diariamente? [Se for "han-
    seníase," então]: fora de hanseníase?

Do you feel there is enough food for you and your family on a daily basis?
Você sente que há bastante comida para sua família no dia-a-dia?

Is violence a problem in your community?
Você acha que a violência é um problema na sua comunidade?

APPENDIX B:
PATIENT PROFILES

Following are brief profiles of the patients with whom I conducted formal interviews. Pseudonyms have been created for all patients. The ages given are at the time of the interview, in 1998 or 1999.

Afonso, fifty. Born in Rio de Janeiro. Lives in Duque de Caxias. Married with two children. Welder. Catholic. Completed treatment for multibacillary leprosy.

Alexandre, fifteen. Born in Cascadura. Living with parents in Duque de Caxias, specifically Santa Cruz da Serra. High school student. Igreja Universal. Completed treatment.

Alícia, (age) thirty-nine. Lives in Duque de Caxias. Married with two children. Works in an insecticide factory. Cristão (evangelical Protestant). Completed treatment for multibacillary leprosy.

Beth, nineteen. Born in Rio de Janeiro. Lives in Bonsucesso. Living with boyfriend. No children. Has worked as a nanny (babá) but had applied for a job at a store. Catholic. Completed treatment.

Celso, forty-four. Born in Rio de Janeiro. Lives in Bonsucesso. Married but sleeping in separate rooms. No children. Used to work as an aviation technician at an airline but had to stop because of complications with the disease. Cristão (but has some reservations about his religion). Completed treatment for multibacillary leprosy.

Clarice, in her thirties. Born in Rio de Janeiro. Father from Rio, mother from Salvador. Lives in Estácio. No children. Works in telecommunications. Catholic. Just getting tested for Hansen's disease and finding out more about it.

Cláudio, twenty-one. Born in Rio de Janeiro. Lives in Anchieta with parents. Has one child. Student. Was interning in a hospital in the pathology lab before he was diagnosed. Cristão. In treatment for paucibacillary leprosy.

Daniela, nineteen. Born in Rio de Janeiro. Lives in Campos Elíseos, Duque de Caxias. Father from Minas Gerais. Not married, no children. Lives at home with parents. Helps at home and could not get a job because of her appearance, she said. Assembly of God. Completed treatment in 1996.

Denilda, forty-nine. Born in Minas Gerais. Lives in Realengo. Married with two children. Domestic worker. Catholic. Completed treatment.

Denise, twenty-seven. Born in Rio de Janeiro. Lives in Oxim (near Nova Iguaçu). Married with three children. Does not work. Igreja Universal. Completed treatment.

Elena, forty-eight. Has lived in Rio de Janeiro since she was a baby. Parents from Macaé. Lives in Sara Coruna. Married with three children. Prepare lunches as at a high school. Catholic.

Elise, twenty-three. Born in Rio de Janeiro. Lives in Bangu. Not married. Hospitalized several times because of leprosy reaction. Studying accounting. Left school temporarily because of her illness. Assembly of God.

Eugênio, seventy. Born in Portugal. Came to Brazil in 1950 because of poor economic conditions in Portugal. Lives in Nilópolis. Married with a daughter. Son died from a gunshot wound. Currently retired but used to work for a paint company. Catholic. Completed treatment.

Fernando, twenty. Born and living in Belford Roxo. Not married, no children. Serving in the army. Former state karate champion. Baptist. Completed treatment for multibacillary leprosy.

Flávia, forty-seven. Born in Minas Gerais. Lives in Nova Iguaçu. Married with two children. Works at a school. Presbyterian (formerly Catholic). Received final dose for paucibacillary leprosy on day of interview.

Geraldo, thirty-eight. Born in Rio de Janeiro. Living in Nilópolis. Also has HIV and toxoplasmosis but has been taking the drug cocktail for HIV and has not developed symptoms of AIDS. Protestant. Completed treatment for multibacillary leprosy.

Gerson, twenty-three. Born in Ceará. Lives in Sara Coruna. Married with two children. Works at a factory building buses but on leave because of disability. Did not say his religion but says he goes to church occasionally. Completed treatment.

Heloísa, twenty-three. Born in Minas Gerais but moved to Rio de Janeiro with her parents when she was a baby. Married with two children. Housewife. Assembly of God. Still in treatment.

Humberto, fifty (wife present at interview). Born in Minas Gerais. Lives in Ramos. Married with four children. Currently out of work but usually works as a driver of a private car. Evangelical.

Inés, forty-two. Born in Minas Gerais. Came to Rio de Janeiro at age thirteen. Lives in Vilar dos Teles. Worked as *faxineira* (domestic worker who does primarily cleaning tasks) but now can't work because of illness. Married with three children. Says she is Catholic but attends a Baptist church.

Ivan, fifty-five (wife present at interview). Born in João Pessoa, Paraíba. Living in Jacarezinho. Banker for twenty-six years who is currently out of work because of leprosy disability. Also recently diagnosed with diabetes. Baptist. In treatment for multibacillary leprosy.

Jacira, forty-five. Born in Rio de Janeiro. Living in Realengo. Widow with four children. Works as a cleaning woman. Unsure of religion, but believes in God (son is Evangelical, daughter is a member of an Afro-Brazilian religion). Completed treatment.

Janete, forty-one. Born in Bonsucesso. Lives in Belford Roxo. Married with one child. Works in a clothing factory. Baptist. Completed treatment for paucibacillary leprosy.

Laura, in her forties. Born in Natal, but moved to Rio twenty years ago. Married with two children. Lives in Vila do Pinheiro. Formerly a cashier at a medical research center. Catholic. Completed treatment.

Lorenzo, forty-two. Lives in Nilópolis. Married with two sons. Mechanic for a major airline. Assembly of God. Had not yet received the definitive diagnosis of leprosy, although he had gone through several weeks of tests. Anxious about the diagnosis and how he will support his family.

Marilene, twenty-four. Born in Rio de Janeiro. Lives in Campo Grande. Not married. Severe reactions. Came to the clinic, where I interviewed her specifically for free pentoxifiline. University student of Portuguese literature. Catholic. Completed treatment for multibacillary leprosy.

Manoel, thirty. Born in São João de Meriti. Lives on the Ilha do Governador. Became very sick before diagnosis. Partner (not an official marriage) left him after he became sick. Abandoned by friends as well. Used to do *biscate* (odd jobs)—selling things in the favelas; still sells occasionally but not often because of disability; does some painting now (buildings). Unsure of religion. Completed treatment for multibacillary leprosy.

Nelson, twenty-eight. Born in Botafogo, Rio de Janeiro. Lives in Vilar dos Teres (in the Baixada Fluminense). Works in metallurgy. *Cristão.* Completed treatment for multibacillary leprosy.

Nilza, forty. Born in Pará. Came to Rio with her mother when she was young. Lives in Nova Iguaçu. Separated from husband. Two children. Currently out of work. Just began treatment for paucibacillary leprosy.

Odete, thirteen (interview questions about Odete were primarily answered by her older sister). Born in Rio de Janeiro. Lives in Nova Iguaçu with parents. Her school tried to forbid her to attend. Unsure about religion (sister is Cristão, mother is Catholic). In treatment.

Pamela, forty-eight. Born in Espírito Santo. Living in Queimados. Single. No children. Currently out of work, surviving on a government pension. Igreja Universal (formerly Catholic). Completed treatment.

Patrícia, twenty-two. Born in Rio de Janeiro. Living in Penha. Not married, no children. Lives with parents. Works as a cashier at the bakery where her father works (had to change jobs to make appointments). Depression and weight gain with reaction problems/prednisone. Completed treatment for multibacillary leprosy.

Regina, thirty-four. Born in Rio de Janeiro. Mother from Rio, father from Minas Gerais. Lives on the Ilha do Governador. Married with two children. Domestic worker in the past. Currently unemployed. Catholic.

Renata, thirty-six. Born in Rio de Janeiro. Married with three children. Unemployed. Used to work in a hospital. Husband had leprosy but no reactions or complications and so is very unsupportive. Catholic. Completed treatment for multibacillary leprosy.

Roberto, forty. Born in Natal. Married with two children. Lives in Campo Grande. Hospitalized twice with reactions. Electrician. Catholic.

Sérgio, twenty-seven. Born in Rio de Janeiro. Parents from Minas Gerais. Lives in Bonsucesso now. Not married, no children. Painter. Served in military in the past. Catholic. Completed treatment.

Sônia, forty-four. Born in Rio de Janeiro. Living in Niterói. Divorced. Unable to work because of the disease. Used to be a domestic worker. Occasionally volunteers for MORHAN. Evangelical. Completed treatment.

Vicente, seventeen. Born in Rio de Janeiro. Lives with family in São João de Meriti. Works in construction/odd jobs. Assembly of God.

Walter, twenty-eight. Born in Rio de Janeiro. Father from Pernambuco, mother from Paraná. Lives in Bonsucesso. Not married, no children. Currently unemployed. Used to work in metallurgy. Evangelical.

Wilson, thirty-six (wife present at interview). Born in Arauão (interior of the state of Rio de Janeiro). Living in the city. Married, no children. Works as an artisan, making baskets. Catholic.

Xavier, thirty-two. Born in Rio de Janeiro. Lives with wife and son. His brothers were killed in gang- or police-related violence; they used to rob city buses. Works as a security guard in a Leblon apartment complex. Catholic. Completed treatment.

Ximena, fifty. Born in Ceará. Came to Rio in the 1970s. Lives in Nova Iguaçu. Worked as a nurse in Ceará; took a job as a domestic worker in Rio, but stopped working after marriage. Catholic. Completed treatment.

Zé, fifty. Born in Rio de Janeiro. Father from Pernambuco, mother from Minas Gerais. Lives in Campos Elísios. Divorced and now "*amigada*" (living with someone). Four children, ten grandchildren. Plumber. Catholic. Completed treatment.

REFERENCE LIST

Ahearn, L. 2001. Language and Agency. *Annual Review of Anthropology* 30:109–137.

Altieri, A. 2001. The Value of a Diploma in Prison. *Brazzil Magazine*, March 18. http://www.brazzil.com/p18mar01.htm (accessed November 20, 2005).

Alves, D., and C. Timmins. 2003. Social Exclusion and the Two-Tiered Healthcare System in Brazil. In *Who's In and Who's Out: Social Exclusion in Latin America*, ed. J. Behrman, A. Gaviria, and M. Szekely, 45–72. Washington, D.C.: Inter-American Development Bank.

American Leprosy Missions Brazil. 2005. História de Vida: J.R.S. http://www.almbrasil.com.br/historia13.htm (accessed December 11, 2005).

Andaló, P. 2003. Love, Tears, Betrayal . . . and Public Health Messages. *Perspectives in Health Magazine: The Magazine of the Pan American Health Organization* 8(2). http://www.paho.org/English/DD/PIN/Number17_article2_1.htm (accessed March 2, 2005).

Andrade, M. 1997. A Cura Como Conceito Vivido: A Ex-Sistir das Pessoas Que Se Submeteram a Poliquimioterapia Para Tratamento da Hanseníase. PhD diss., Universidade Federal do Rio de Janeiro, Centro de Ciências da Saúde, Escola de Enfermagem Ana Nery.

Andrade, V. and M. Virmond. 2004. Partnership and Decentralization: A New Approach to Eliminating Leprosy in Brazil. http://www.novartisfoundation.com/en/projects/access_health/leprosy/diagnosis/brazil_partnership_ decentralization.htm#encouraging_results (accessed June 1, 2004).

Astor, M. 1998. Brazil's Energetic Pop Star Priest Taking the Country by Storm. Associated Press story. *Laredo Morning Times*, December 20, p. 18A.

———. 2004. Pop Goes the Priest. Associated Press story. *Halifax Herald Limited*, March 27: n.p.

Bárbara, L., A. Burman, H. Medeiros, M. Camargo, and M. Collins, eds. 1989. *Michaelis Pequeno Dicionário. Inglês-Português, Português- Inglês*. São Paulo: Companhia Melhoramentos de São Paulo.

Bar-Ilan, M. 2002. Between Magic and Religion: Sympathetic Magic in the World of the Sages of the Misnah and Torah. *Review of Rabbinic Studies* 5(3): 383–399.

Barrett, R. 2005. Self-Mortification and the Stigma of Leprosy in Northern India. *Medical Anthropology Quarterly* 19(2): 216–230.

Bastide, R. 1978. *O Candomblé da Bahia (Rito Nago)*. Trans. M.I.P. Queiroz. São Paulo: Companhia Editora Nacional.

Bernard, H. R. 2002. *Research Methods in Anthropology*. Walnut Creek, Calif.: Altamira Press.

Biehl, J. 2004. Life of the Mind: The Interface of Psychopharmaceuticals, Domestic Economies, and Social Abandonment. *American Ethnologist* 31(4): 475–496.

Bittencourt, M. 1999. Médicos Ignoram Plantão. *Jornal do Brasil*, March 29, p. 17.

Bochenek, M., and F. Delgado. 2005. In the Dark: Hidden Abuses against Detained Youths in Rio de Janeiro. New York: Human Rights Watch.

Bourdieu, P. 1986. The Forms of Capital. In *Handbook of Theory and Research for the Sociology of Education*, ed. J. G. Richardson, 241–258. New York: Greenwood Press.

Bourgois, P. 1995. *In Search of Respect: Selling Crack in El Barrio*. Cambridge: Cambridge University Press.

Brand, P., and P. Yancey. 1993. *Pain: The Gift Nobody Wants*. New York: HarperCollins.

Briggs, C. 1986. *Learning How to Ask: A Sociolinguistic Appraisal of the Role of the Interview in Social Science Research*. Cambridge: Cambridge University Press.

Brody, S. 1974. *The Disease of the Soul: Leprosy in Medieval Literature*. Ithaca, N.Y.: Cornell University Press.

Bührer-Sékula, S., H. L. Smits, G. C. Gussenhoven, J. Van Leeuwen, S. Amador, T. Fujiwara, P. R. Klatser, and L. Oskam. 2003. Simple and Fast Lateral Flow Test for Classification of Leprosy Patients and Identification of Contacts with High Risk of Developing Leprosy. *Journal of Clinical Microbiology* 41(5): 1991–1995.

Caprara, A.1998. Médico Ferido: Omolu nos Labirintos da Doença. In *Antropologia da Saúde: Traçando Identidade e Explorando Fronteiras*, ed. P. C. Alves and M. C. Rabelo, 123–138. Rio de Janeiro:Editora Fiocruz.

Carciániga, C., and S. Herselman. 1999. Leprosy and Anthropological Insights. *South African Journal of Ethnology* 22(4): 157–171.

Cézar, J. 2004. Brazil Sees Death Squad in Homeless Massacre. *Brazzil Magazine*, August 1. http://www.brazzil.com/content/view/2069/51 (accessed September 1, 2006).

Chesnut, R. A. 1997. *Born Again in Brazil: The Pentecostal Boom and the Pathogens of Poverty*. New Brunswick, N.J.: Rutgers University Press.

Claro, L. 1995. *Hanseníase: Representações Sobre a Doença*. Rio de Janeiro: Fundação Oswaldo Cruz.

Correio Braziliense. 1995. 'Lepra' é Censurada em Documento Oficial. *Correio Braziliense*, March 31, 1995 (taken from clippings or Recortes of the Ministério da Sáude, Assessória de Comunicação Social, Brasília, n.p.).

Country-data.com. 1997. Brazil: Conscription. http://www.country-data.com/cgi-bin/query/r-1804.html (accessed November 20, 2005).

Crandon-Malamud, L. 1993. *From the Fat of Our Souls: Social Change, Political Process, and Medical Pluralism in Bolivia*. Berkeley: University of California Press.

Cunha, S., L. Rodrigues, and N. Duppre. 2004. Current Strategy for Leprosy Control in Brazil: Time to Pursue Alternative Preventive Strategies? *Revista Panamericana de Salud Pública* 16(5): 362–365.

Cutler, J., dir. 1993. *Thalidomide: Still With Us* (video production) (alternate title: *Thalidomide: The Drug that Came Back*). Leeds, England: Yorkshire Television.

Deutsche-Welle. 2004. Brazil: Getting Children Back to School. http://www.dw-world.de/dw/article/0,1564,1103646,00.html (accessed February 1, 2007).

Douglas, M.1966. *Purity and Danger: An Analysis of Concepts of Pollution and Taboo*. New York: Praeger.

————.1991. Witchcraft and Leprosy: Two Strategies of Exclusion. *Man* 26(4): 723–736.

Draffen, A., C. McAsey, L. Pinheiro, and R. Jones. 1996. *Brazil: A Lonely Planet Travel Survival Kit.* Oakland, Calif.: Lonely Planet.

Dunn, C. 2001. *Brutality Garden: Tropicália and the Emergence of a Brazilian Counterculture.* Chapel Hill: University of North Carolina Press.

Duran, S.M.O. 1995. SER-Um Analisador Histórico: A Demanda de Atendimento Num *Ambulatório da Rede Pública.* Monograph presented to the postgraduate course Lato Sensu: Psychological Theories and Practices in Public Institutions—Ambulatory Area—A Transdisciplinary Focus of Clinical Practice, as part of the requirements toward the title of Specialist. Niterói, Brazil: Universidade Federal Fluminense.

Eisenberg, L. 1977. Disease and Illness: Distinctions between Professional and Popular Ideas of Sickness. *Culture, Medicine, and Psychiatry* 1(1): 9–23.

Farmer, P. 1993. *AIDS and Accusation: Haiti and the Geography of Blame.* Berkeley: University of California Press.

————. 1999. *Infections and Inequalities: The Modern Plagues.* Berkeley: University of California Press.

————. 2004. An Anthropology of Structural Violence. *Current Anthropology* 45(3): 305–325.

Farmer, P., S. Robin, S. Ramilus, and J. Kim. 1991. Tuberculosis, Poverty, and 'Compliance': Lessons from Rural Haiti. *Seminars in Respiratory Infections* 6(4): 254–260.

Feenstra, P. 2003. 'Elimination' of Leprosy and the Need to Sustain Leprosy Services, Expectations, Predictions, and Reality. *International Journal of Leprosy* 71(3): 248–256.

Feeny, P. 1964. *The Fight against Leprosy.* London: Elek Books.

Filho, A. 2005. Populismo Revisitado. http://www.terra.com.br/istoe/1849/brasil/1849_populismo_revisitado.htm (accessed September 23, 2005).

Fine, P., I. Carneiro, J. Milstien, C. Clements. 1999. Issues Related to the Use of BCG Vaccine in Immunization Programs: A Discussion Document. Geneva, Switzerland: Department of Vaccines and Biologicals, World Health Organization. http://www.who.int/vaccines-documents/DocsPDF99/www9943.pdf (accessed November 19, 2005).

Fiori, M. 2004. Only Bosses Happy with Brazil's New Minimum Wage. *Brazzil Magazine,* April 2004. http://www.brazzil.com/2004/html/articles/apr04/p140apr04.htm (accessed October 3, 2004).

Fontoura, A. A., A.H.F. Barcelos, and V. T. Borges. 2003. Revealing a History of Exclusion: The Experience at Hospital-Colônia Itapuã Data and Research Center. *História, Ciências, Saúde—Manguinhos* 10(sup. 1): 397–414.

Foster, G. 1953. What Is Folk Culture? *American Anthropologist* 55(2), Part 1: 159–173.

————.1976. Disease Etiologies in Nonwestern Medical Systems. *American Anthropologist* 78(4): 773–782.

Foucault, M. 1988. *Madness and Civilization: A History of Insanity in the Age of Reason.* New York: Vintage Books.

————.1994. *The Birth of the Clinic: An Archaeology of Medical Perception.* New York: Vintage Books.

Frazer, J. 1922. *The Golden Bough: A Study in Magic and Religion.* New York: Macmillan.

Gabbay, J. 1982. Asthma Attacked: Tactics for the Reconstruction of a Disease Concept. In *The Problem of Medical Knowledge*, ed. P. Wright and A. Treacher, 23–48. Edinburgh: Edinburgh University Press.

Galtung, J. 1969. Violence, Peace, and Peace Research. *Journal of Peace Research* 6(3): 167–191.

Garbarino, M. 1977. *Sociocultural Theory in Anthropology: A Short History*. Prospect Heights, Ill.: Waveland Press.

Gerência de Dermatologia Sanitária. 1998. *Casos de Abandono*. Rio de Janeiro: Gerência de Dermatologia Sanitária/CDT/SSC/SMS.

Goertzel, T. 2003. So, This Is Lula? *Brazzil Magazine*, January. http://www.brazzil. com/p118jan03.htm (accessed June 5, 2005).

Goffman, E. 1963. Stigma: *Notes on the Management of Spoiled Identity*. Englewood Cliffs, N.J.: Prentice-Hall.

Goldstein, D. 2003. *Laughter out of Place: Race, Class, Violence, and Sexuality in a Rio Shantytown*. Berkeley: University of California Press.

Good, B. and M. DelVecchio-Good. 1993. "'Learning Medicine': The Constructing of Medical Knowledge at Harvard Medical School. In *Knowledge, Power, and Practice: The Anthropology of Medicine in Everyday Life*, ed. S. Lindenbaum and M. Lock, 81–107. Berkeley and Los Angeles: University of California Press.

Goulart, I.M.B, G. L. Arbex, M. H. Carneiro, M. S. Rodrigues, and R. Gadia. 2002. Adverse Effects of Multidrug Therapy in Leprosy Patients: A Five-Year Survey at a Health Center of the Federal University of Uberlândia. *Revista da Sociedade Brasileira de Medicina Tropical* 35(5): 453–460.

Graham, R. 1999. Free African Brazilians and the State in Slavery Times. In *Racial Politics in Contemporary Brazil*, ed. M. Hanchard, 30–58. Durham, N.C: Duke University Press.

Greene, J. 2004. An Ethnography of Nonadherence: Culture, Poverty, and Tuberculosis in Urban Bolivia. *Culture, Medicine, and Psychiatry* 28(3): 401–425.

Greenfield, S. 1999. Hypnosis and Trance Induction in the Surgeries of Brazilian Spiritist Healer-Mediums. In *Across the Boundaries of Belief: Contemporary Issues in the Anthropology of Religion*, ed. M. Klauss and M. Weisgrau, 211–226. Boulder, Colo.: Westview Press.

Gregg, J. 2003. *Virtually Virgins: Sexual Strategies and Cervical Cancer in Recife, Brazil*. Stanford, Calif.: Stanford University Press.

Grimm, D. 2005. Global Spread of Leprosy Tied to Human Migration. *Science* 308: 936–937.

Gussow, Z. 1989. *Leprosy, Racism, and Public Health*. Boulder, Colo.: Westview Press.

Gwei-Djen, L., and J. Needham. 1967. Records of Diseases in Ancient China. In *Diseases in Antiquity*, ed. D. Brothwell, 222–237. Springfield, Ill.: Charles C. Thomas Publishers.

Hahn, R. 1998. The Nocebo Phenomenon: Concept, Evidence, and Implications for Public Health. In *Understanding and Applying Medical Anthropology*, ed. by P. Brown, 138–143. Mountainview, Calif.: Mayfield Publishing.

Harris, M. 1975. *Cows, Pigs, Wars, and Witches: The Riddles of Culture*. New York: Vintage Books.

———.1980. *Cultural Materialism: The Struggle for a Science of Culture*. New York: Random House.

Harvard School of Public Health. 2005. Food Pyramids. http://www.hsph.harvard. edu/nutritionsource/pyramids.html (accessed September 3, 2005).

Hassel, J. 1997. Campaign to Wipe out Leprosy Criticized. *New Orleans Times Picayune*, July 13: A-8.

Hastings, R. 1985. *Leprosy*. New York: Churchill Livingstone.

Heidegger, M. 1962. *Being and Time*. New York: Harper & Row.

HostelPlanet.com. 2004. Favela Hostel, Rio de Janeiro Brazil. http://www.hostelplanet.com/hostelplanet.com/hostel.php/HostelNumber.10186 (accessed March 2, 2005).

Instituto Brasileiro de Geografia e Estatística (IBGE).2000. Domicílios por Condição de Saneamento e Luz Eléctrica. Pesquisa Nacional por Amostra de Domicílios. Microdados: Rio de Janeiro, 1999. http://www.ibge.gov.br/ (accessed August 12, 2005).

———.2005. IBGE-Cidades/Rio de Janeiro. http://www.ibge.gov.br/cidadesat/ (accessed August 25, 2005).

Instituto de Pesquisa Histórica e Análises Sociais da Baixada Fluminense (IPAHB). 2004. São João de Meriti. http://www.broncalivre.com.br/sjm.html (accessed September 28, 2004).

Jewison, N., dir. 1973. *Jesus Christ Superstar*. Universal City, Calif.: Universal Pictures.

Jornal do Brasil (no author cited). 1999. Postos Enfrentam Falta de Remédios. *Jornal do Brasil*. July 22, p. 19.

Justice, J. 1995. The Politics of Infectious Diseases: A Case Study of Leprosy and Its Elimination. Paper presented at 94th annual meeting of the American Anthropological Association, Washington, D.C., November 17.

Kapferer, B. 1983. *A Celebration of Demons: Exorcism and Aesthetics of Healing in Sri Lanka*. Bloomington: Indiana University Press.

Karasch, M. 1987. *Slave Life in Rio de Janeiro: 1808–1850*. Princeton, N.J.: Princeton University Press.

Karonga Prevention Trial Group. 1996. *The Lancet* 348(9019): 17–24.

Keenan, P., M. Jacobson, R. Soleymani, M. Mayes, M. Stress, and D. Yaldoo. 1996. The Effect on Memory of Chronic Prednisone Treatment in Patients with Systemic Disease. *Neurology* 47(6): 1396–1402.

Kerr-Pontes, L., A. Montenegro, M. Barreto, G. Werneck, and H. Feldmeier. 2004. Inequality and Leprosy in Northeast Brazil: An Ecological Study. *International Journal of Epidemiology* 33(2): 262–269.

Kleinman, A.1980. *Patients and Healers in the Context of Culture*. Berkeley: University of California Press.

———.1988. *The Illness Narratives: Suffering, Healing, and the Human Condition*. New York: Basic Books.

Kloss, J. 1988. *Back to Eden*. Rev. and exp. 2nd ed. Loma Linda, Calif.: Back to Eden Books.

Kottak, C. 2004. *Window on Humanity*. Columbus, Ohio: McGraw-Hill.

Kottak, C., and K. Kozaitis. 2003. *On Being Different*. Columbus, Ohio: McGraw-Hill.

Kroeger, K. 2003. AIDS Rumors, Imaginary Enemies, and the Body Politic in Indonesia. *American Ethnologist* 30(2): 243–257.

Lambert, J. 1978 (1943). *Os Dois Brasis*. São Paulo: Companhia Editora Nacional.

Lemos, S. 2003. The Effect of the Minimum Wage on Prices in Brazil. Discussion paper 04–01, *Discussion Papers in Economics*. Department of Economics, University College, London. http://www.econ.ucl.ac.uk/papers/working_paper_series/0401.pdf (accessed September 5, 2005).

Lesser, J. 1999. *Negotiating National Identities: Immigrants, Minorities, and the Struggle for Ethnicity in Brazil*. Durham, N.C.: Duke University Press.

Lewis, G. 1993. Double Standards of Treatment Evaluation. In *Knowledge, Power, and Practice: The Anthropology of Medicine in Everyday Life*, ed. S. Lindenbaum and M. Lock, 189–218. Berkeley: University of California Press.

Linger, D. 1992. *Dangerous Encounters: Meanings of Violence in a Brazilian City*. Stanford, Calif.: Stanford University Press.

Lisboa, A. 1932. *Pela Pátria, Contra a Lepra, O Mais Perigoso Dos Seus Inimigos*. Rio de Janeiro: São Benedicto.

Lockwood, D. 2004. Commentary: Poverty and Leprosy. *International Journal of Epidemiology* 33(2): 269–270.

Lockwood, D., and B. Kumar. 2004. Treatment of Leprosy: The Evidence Base for Newer Drug Combinations and Shorter Regimens in Weak. *British Medical Journal* 328:1447–1448.

Mange, P. 1992. Hansen and His Discovery of Mycobacterium leprae. *The Star* September/October:5–8.

Marcus, G. 1995. Ethnography in/of the World System. *Annual Review of Anthropology* 24: 95–117.

Mariner, J., and J. Cavallaro. 1998. *Behind Bars in Brazil*. New York: Human Rights Watch.

Martin, B. 1950. *Miracle at Carville*. Garden City, N.Y.: Doubleday.

Martin, E. 1994. *Flexible Bodies: The Role of Immunity in American Culture from the Days of Polio to the Age of AIDS*. Boston: Beacon Press.

Mattoso, K. 1986. *To Be a Slave in Brazil: 1550–1888*. Trans. A. Goldhammer. New Brunswick, N.J.: Rutgers University Press.

Meirelles, F., and K. Lund, dirs. *Cidade de Deus*. Rio de Janeiro: 02 Filmes.

Ministério de Saúde (Brazilian Ministry of Health). 1994. *Guia de Controle da Hanseníase*. Brasília: Fundação Nacional da Saúde.

———.2005. "Farmácia Popular do Brasil." http://dtr2002.saude.gov.br/farmacia popular/ (accessed September 24, 2005).

Mintz, S. 1954. Brief Communications on Redfield and Foster. *American Anthropologist* 56(1): 87–92.

———.1985. *Sweetness and Power: The Place of Sugar in Modern History*. New York: Viking Press.

Monteiro, M. 2004. Do Estuque ao Tijolo. Favela Tem Memória/Viva Rio. http://www.favelatemmemoria.com.br/publique/cgi/cgilua.exe/sys/start.htm?from%5Finfo%5Findex=11&infoid=71&sid=7 (accessed August 26, 2005).

Muslim Student Association–University of Southern California (MSA-USC). 2002. MSA-USC Hadith Database. http://www.usc.edu/dept/MSA/reference/search hadith.html (accessed September 15, 2002).

Nascimento, G. 2005. As Contas Secretas da Igreja Universal. http://www.terra.com.br/istoe/1858/brasil/1858_as_contas_secretas_da_igreja_universal.htm (accessed December 15, 2005).

Neufeldt, V., and D. Guralink, eds. 1988. *Webster's New World Dictionary of American English*. 3rd college ed. New York: Webster's New World.

Neuwirth, R. 2004. *Shadow Cities: A Billion Squatters, A New Urban World*. New York: Routledge.

Neves, F. 2003. Five Million Kids Still Working in Brazil. *Brazzil Magazine*, October 1. http://www.brazzil.com/2003/html/news/articles/oct03/p117oct03.htm (accessed October 3, 2004).

Nguyen, L. N., J. L. Cartel, and J. H. Grosset. 2000. Chemoprophylaxis of Leprosy in the Southern Marquesas with a Single 25 mg/kg Dose of Rifampicin: Results after 10 Years. *Leprosy Review* 71 (4): Suppl. S33–36.

Oliveira, M.A.O., J.A.Z. Bermudez, and A.C.M. Souza. 1999. Talidomida no Brasil: Vigilância com Responsibilidade Compartilhada? *Cadernos de Saúde Pública* 15(1): 99–112.

Oliveira, M. H. 1997. The Effects of Leprosy on Men and Women: A Gender Study. *Gender and Tropical Diseases* (paper series). Geneva: UNDP/World Bank/WHO Special Programme for Research and Training in Tropical Diseases (TDR).

Oliveira, M.L.W., C. M. Mendes, R. T. Tardin, M. D. Cunha, Â. Arruda. 2003. A Representação Social da Hanseníase, Trinta Anos Após a Substituição da Terminologia 'Lepra' no Brasil. *História, Ciências, Saúde—Manguinhos* 10(sup. 1): 41–48.

Ortner, D., and W. Putschar. 1985. *Identification of Pathological Conditions in Human Skeletal Remains.* Washington, D.C.: Smithsonian Institution Press.

Padilha, J., and F. Lacerda, dir. 2002. *Ônibus 174.* Rio de Janeiro: Zazen Produções.

Page, J. 1995. *The Brazilians.* New York: Addison-Wesley Publishing.

Pannikar, V. 1985. *History of Leprosy.* Karigiri, India: KLEP Series Karigiri.

Parker, R., and P. Aggleton. 2003. HIV and AIDS-related Stigma and Discrimination: A Conceptual Framework and Implication for Action. *Social Science and Medicine* 57(1): 13–24.

Penglase, B. 1994. *Final Justice: Police and Death Squad Homicides of Adolescents in Brazil.* New York: Human Rights Watch.

Pereira, R. 1996. *Hanseníase na Mulher: Suas Representações no Contexto Familiar.* Rio de Janeiro: Fundação Oswaldo Cruz.

Perlman, J. 1976. *The Myth of Marginality: Urban Poverty and Politics in Rio de Janeiro.* Berkeley: University of California Press.

Perri, A., and S. Hsu. 2003. A Review of Thalidomide's History and Current Dermatological Applications. *Dermatology Online Journal* 9(3): 5.

Pontes, F., and S. Schmidt. 2001. A Invasão Silenciosa das Favelas. Originally in *Globo* newspaper, January 28, 2001. http://hps.infolink.com.br/peco/cbo10128.htm (accessed April 16, 2005).

Queiroz, M., and M. Puntel. 1997. *A Endemia Hansênica: Uma Perspectiva Multidisciplinar.* Rio de Janeiro: Editora Fiocruz.

Quintão, E., ed. 1998. *Como Curar Com Remédios Caseiros,* vol. 2. Rio de Janeiro: AKS Editora.

Rádio Viva News. 2007. Brasil: Salário Mínimo Será $408,90 em 2008. http://www.radioviva.com.br/viva890/noticia.php?noticia=19583 (accessed January 4, 2008).

Rao, S., V. Garole, S. Walawalkar, S. Khot, and N. Karandikar. 1996. Gender Differentials in the Social Impact of Leprosy. *Leprosy Review* 67(3): 190–199.

Rede Globo Rio de Janeiro. 1998. Local news broadcast, November 19.

Redfield, R. 1930. *Tepotlzán: A Mexican Village.* Chicago: University of Chicago Press.

———.1940. The Folk Society and Culture. *American Journal of Sociology* 45(5): 731–742.

Ribeiro, R. 2003. Pensar o Brasil. *O Mundo em Português* 41 (February). http://www.ieei.pt/publicacoes/exemplar.php?exemplar=55 (accessed November 1, 2005).

Ryerson, W. 2005. The Effectiveness of Entertainment Mass Media in Changing Behavior. http://www.populationmedia.org/programs/effectiv.html (accessed November 20, 2005). Saunderson, P. 2002. *How to Recognise and Manage Leprosy*

Reactions. London: The International Federation of Anti-Leprosy Associations (ILEP).

Sandreczki, M. 1889. A Study on Leprosy. *The Lancet*, August 31, cited in Tebb 1893, no page number given.

Sarti, C. 1995. Morality and Transgression among Brazilian Poor Families: Exploring Ambiguities. In *The Brazilian Puzzle: Culture on the Borderlands of the Western World*, ed. D. Hess and R. Da Matta., 114–133. New York: Columbia University Press.

Scheper-Hughes, N. 1992. *Death without Weeping: The Violence of Everyday Life in Brazil*. Berkeley: University of California Press.

Scheper-Hughes, N., and M. Lock. 1987. The Mindful Body: A Prolegomenon to a Future Work in Medical Anthropology. *Medical Anthropology Quarterly* 1(1):6–41.

Scollard, D. 2004. Classification of Leprosy: A Full Color Spectrum or Black and White? *International Journal of Leprosy and other Mycobacterial Diseases* 72(2):166–168.

———.2005. Leprosy Research Declines, But Most of the Basic Questions Remain Unanswered (Editorial). *International Journal of Leprosy and Other Mycobacterial Diseases* 73(1): 25–27.

Secretaria Municipal de Saúde do Rio de Janeiro. 1997. *Oportunidades Perdidas de Diagnóstico e Tratamento da Hanseníase* (1-page document). Rio de Janeiro: Gerência de Dermatologia Sanitária.

Segerstrom, S., and G. Miller. 2004. Psychological Stress and the Human Immune System: A Meta-Analytic Study of 30 Years of Inquiry. *Psychological Bulletin* 130(4): 601–630.

Silva, S., and H. Tassara. 1996. *Fruit in Brazil*. São Paulo: Empresa das Artes.

Sistema Único de Saúde. 2004. Ô Que É O SUS? http://www.sespa.pa.gov.br/Sus/Sus/sus_oquee.htm (accessed: October 8, 2004).

Skillicorn, K. 1998. http://forums.delphi.com/lepforum/ (accessed March 1, 1998).

Skinses, O. 1964. Leprosy in Society. *Leprosy Review* 35(1): 13–15.

Skolnik, R., F. Agueh, J. Justice, and M. Lechat. 2003. *Independent Evaluation of the Global Alliance for the Elimination of Leprosy*. Geneva: World Health Organization.

Smith, C., and W. Smith. 2000. Chemoprophylaxis Is Effective in the Prevention of Leprosy in Endemic Countries: A Systematic Review and Meta-Analysis. *Journal of Infection* 41(2): 137–142.

Smith, T. H. 2003. A Monument to Lazarus: The Leprosy Hospital of Rio de Janeiro. *História, Ciências, Saúde—Manguinhos* 10(sup. 1): 143–160.

———. 2002. Leprosy in the New World: Leprosy Hospitals in Colonial Spanish America. Paper presented at the History of Leprosy–Microbiol Exchanges Symposium at the XVI International Leprosy Congress, Salvador, Brazil, August 7.

Sontag, S. 1990. *Illness as Metaphor and AIDS and Its Metaphors*. New York: Doubleday.

Souza-Araújo, H.C.S. 1946. *História da Lepra no Brasil*. Vol.1, *Períodos Colonial e Monárquico (1500–1889)*. Rio de Janeiro: Imprensa Nacional.

———. 1948. *História da Lepra no Brasil*. Vol. 2, *Período Republicano (1889–1946)*. Rio de Janeiro: Imprensa Nacional.

Staples, J. 2004. Delineating Disease: Self-Management of Leprosy Identities in South India. *Medical Anthropology* 23(1): 68–89.

Stein, S., and L. Blochman. 1963. *Alone No Longer*. New York: Funk & Wagnalls.

Talhari, S., and R. Neves. 1997. *Dermatologia Tropical: Hanseníase*. 3rd ed. Manaus, Brazil: Gráfica Tropical.

Tebb, W. 1893. *Leprosy and Vaccination*. London: Swan Sonnenschein. http://www.whale.to/v/tebb/leprosy.html (accessed February 1, 2003).

Tesh, S., and E. Paes-Machado. 2004. Sewers, Garbage, and Environmentalism in Brazil. *Journal of Environment and Development* 13(1): 42–72.

Thielen, E., and L. O. Coimbra. 1992. (video) *Iarere: Hanseníase e Mentalidades em Rio De Janeiro*. Rio de Janeiro: Casa de Oswaldo Cruz.

Trautman, J. 1989. Epidemiological Aspects of Hansen's Disease (HD). *The Star* 49(2): n.p.

Vaughan, M. 1991. *Curing Their Ills: Colonial Power and African Illness*. Stanford, Calif.: Stanford University Press.

Veloso, C. 1967. Alegria, Alegria (song). Single album: *Alegria alegria*. Philips Records.

———. 2002. Tropical Truth: A Story of Music and Revolution in Brazil. New York: Alfred A. Knopf.

Viola, P., and H. B. Carvalho. 1996. Timoneiro (song). *Bebadosamba*. RCA.

VivaRio. 2005. Rumo à Zona Oeste. Favela Tem Memória website. http://www.vivafavela.com.br/frame.asp?url=http://www.favelatemmemoria.com.br/publique/cgi/cgilua.exe/sys/start.htm?sid=7&infoid=104 (accessed August 26, 2005).

Voeks, R. 1997. *Sacred Leaves of Candomblé: African Magic, Medicine, and Religion in Brazil*. Austin: University of Texas Press.

Wagley, C. 1971. *An Introduction to Brazil*. Rev. ed. New York: Columbia University Press.

———. 1995. A Most Personal People. In *Brazilian Mosaic: Portraits of a Diverse People and Culture*, ed. G. H. Summ, 148–153. Wilmington, Del.: Scholarly Resources.

Wallerstein, I. 1974. *The Modern World System: Capitalist Agriculture and the Origins of the European World Economy in the Sixteenth Century*. New York: Academic Press.

Ward, P. (prod.). 1999. *Banished: Living with Leprosy* (video). Great Falls, Va.: Ward & Associates.

Weizman, S. 2003. Ancient Leper's Bones Found in Jerusalem. Associated Press story from December 31, 2003. http://msnbc.msn.com/id/3849407/ (accessed February 1, 2004).

White, C. 1996. Physical and Metaphorical Confinement: The Experience of Hansen's Disease (Leprosy) in the United States. *Human Mosaic* 30 (1–2):12–28.

———. 2003. Carville and Curupaiti: Experiences of Confinement and Community. *História, Ciências, Saúde—Manguinhos* 10(sup. 1): 123–142.

———. 2005. Explaining a Complex Disease Process: Talking to Patients about Leprosy in Brazil. *Medical Anthropological Quarterly* 19(3): 310–330.

———. 2007. Iatrogenic Stigma in Outpatient Treatment for Hansen's Disease (Leprosy) in Brazil. *Health Education Research*. Advance Access published on January 17, DOI 10.1093/her/cyl158.

Wolf, E. 1982. *Europe and the People without History*. Berkeley: University of California Press.

Wong, M. L. 2002. Can Social Marketing Be Applied to Leprosy Programmes? *Leprosy Review* 73(4): 308–318.

World Bank. 2002. World Development Index 2002. http://www.infoplease.com/ipa/A0908770.html (accessed August 12, 2005).

World Health Organization. 1997. *A Guide to Eliminating Leprosy as a Public Health Problem.* 2nd ed. Geneva: WHO/Action Programme for the Elimination of Leprosy.

———. 1999. What Are the New Antileprosy Drugs—ROM—Now Available for the Treatment of Leprosy? http://www.who.int/lep/romfaq/frmain.htm (accessed November 1, 2000).

———. 2003. *The Final Push Strategy to Eliminate Leprosy as a Public Health Problem: Questions and Answers.* 2nd ed. Geneva: World Health Organization.

———. 2004. Elimination of Leprosy as a Public Health Problem. http://www.who.int/lep/disease/disease.htm (accessed Feb. 1, 2004).

———. 2005a. Global Leprosy Situation 2005. *Weekly Epidemiological Record* 80(35):289–295. http://www.who.int/lep/Reports/wer8034.pdf (accessed November 20, 2005).

———. 2005b. Global Strategy for Further Reducing the Leprosy Burden and Sustaining Leprosy Control Activities. Geneva: World Health Organization.

———. 2005c. Microbiology of Leprosy: Transmission. http://www.who.int/lep/disease/Microbiology/micro.htm (accessed November 4, 2005).

———. 2005d. The President of Chile and the WHO Director-General Launch Global Health Commission to Tackle the 'Causes Behind the Causes of Ill-Health' News Release, March 18, 2005. *http://www.who.int/mediacentre/news/releases/2005/pr13/en/index.html* (accessed March 24, 2005).

———. 2007a. Leprosy, Fact Sheet No. 101. http://www.who.int/mediacentre/factsheets/fs101/en/print.html (accessed June 1, 2007).

———. 2007b. New Case Detection Trends in Leprosy. http://www.who.int/lep/situation/NCDetection2006.pdf (accessed March 8, 2007).

———. 2007c. Prevalence of Leprosy. *http://www.who.int/lep/situation/prevalence/en/index.html* (accessed June 1, 2007).

World Organization of the Scouting Movement (WOSM). 2005. Scouting and the Fight against Leprosy. http://www.scout.org/wsrc/fs/scoutsleprosy_e.shtml (accessed February 12, 2005).

Wyler, W., dir. 1959. *Ben Hur.* Culver City, Calif.: Metro-Goldwyn-Mayer.

INDEX

A&E network, 2
abandonment of treatment: assumptions
about, 19; drug side effects and, 114–115,
156; house visits to counter, 122–124;
measures to avoid, 187; patient agency
and, 180–181; patients' reasons for, 119–
122; rates of, 118–119; religious impulse
in, 53; self-stigmatization linked to,
145; WHO's recommendations on, 122,
124–125
Afonso (pseud.), 76, 110, 138, 209
Africa: BCG vaccination in, 188; leprosy
stigma in, 132; leprosy transmission
models in, 69; Portuguese slave trade
in, 31; as possible origin of leprosy, 9.
See also specific countries
Afro-Brazilian popular religions: disease
origin explanations in, 73–74; healing
in, 50; home remedies linked to,
80–81; influences on, 49; leprosy cure
in, 78–79; leprosy stigma and, 135;
negative views of, 50
agency: concept of, 26–27; in medical
encounter, 131; patients' expression
of, 179–180; role of, 27–28; structural
constraints on, 183–187. *See also* illness
narratives
Aggleton, Peter, 134
Ahearn, Laura, 26–27
AIDS. *See* HIV/AIDS
alcoholic beverages, 119–120, 166
"Alegria, Alegria" (song), 29–30
Aleijadinho (Little Cripple, Antônio
Francisco Lisboa), 75
aleijado (crippled): use of term, 75
Alexandre (pseud.), 174–177, 209
Alícia (pseud.), 114–115, 143, 209
allergies, 98–99, 173, 197
alta (tall or high; being discharged): use
of term, 16, 115, 167
Amazon region peasants, 32
American Leprosy Missions, 34, 146
Andrade, Marilda, 23–24, 116
Ângela (pseud.), 41–42
Anos Rebeldes (Rebel Years, *novela*), 29–30
anthropology: cognitive, 23; models of
stigma in, 133–134. *See also* medical

anthropology; methodology and
research
antibiotics, 98–99, 111. *See also*
pharmaceutical medicines; *specific
drugs*
área limpo (clean area): use of term, 135
área suja (dirty area): use of term, 135
aroeira *(Schinus terebinthefolius)*, 81
arthritis, 151
Asia: folk models of leprosy in, 59;
leprosy stigma in, 9–10; leprosy
transmission models in, 69;
misdiagnosis of leprosy in, 95–96; as
possible origin of leprosy, 9. *See also
specific countries*
Assembly of God, 173
Associações de Moradores (Residents'
Associations), 36
asthma, 25, 155
azathioprine, 112, 130, 131

Bacillus Camille-Guerin (BCG) vaccine,
187–189
bandidos: construction of, 44–45
Bangladesh: misdiagnosis of leprosy in,
95–96; poverty and leprosy in, 56
Barrett, Ron, 71, 145
BCG (Bacillus Camille-Guerin) vaccine,
187–189
belief systems: naturalistic vs.
personalistic, 66, 73–74. *See also* folk
models; patient explanatory models;
religion
Ben Hur (film), 2
Beth (pseud.), 70, 98–99, 209
Bible: leprosy references in, 9, 59; on sin
and moral transgression, 58; *tzaareth*
(Hebrew term) in, 9, 67
Biehl, João, 185
biomedical models: on asthma, 25;
on cure, 116–117; evangelicals on,
79–80; as fear-inducing, 147; as folk
models, 59–60; on incubation, 176;
leprosy stigma and, 135; on leprosy
transmission, 66–67, 71–72, 73, 169;
military metaphors in, 118; other
models juxtaposed to, 83–84; patients'

ABOUT THE AUTHOR

CASSANDRA WHITE is an assistant professor in the Department of Anthropology at Georgia State University. She currently resides in Decatur, Georgia, with her husband and daughter.